Pharmacology

Concise
Medical
Textbooks

BIOCHEMISTRY
S. P. Datta and J. H. Ottaway
CARDIOLOGY
D. G. Julian
DERMATOLOGY
E. Lipman Cohen and J. S. Pegum
EMBRYOLOGY
M. B. L. Craigmyle
GASTROENTEROLOGY
I. A. D. Bouchier
MEDICAL MICROBIOLOGY
C. G. A. Thomas
OBSTETRICS
J. M. Holmes
OPHTHALMOLOGY
Kenneth Wybar
PAEDIATRICS
John Apley
PATHOLOGY
J. R. Tighe
PHARMACOLOGY
R. G. Penn
PREVENTIVE MEDICINE, COMMUNITY HEALTH AND
SOCIAL SERVICES
J. B. Meredith-Davies
PSYCHIATRY
E. W. Anderson and W. H. Trethowan

Pharmacology

R. G. PENN

M.B., B.CH. (WALES)

Principal Medical Officer, Medicines Division Department of Health and Social Security, Formerly Lecturer in Pharmacology, Charing Cross Hospital Medical School, London

SECOND EDITION

BAILLIÈRE TINDALL ❧ LONDON

A Baillière Tindall book published by
Cassell Ltd, London
35 Red Lion Square, London WC1R 4SG
Sydney, Auckland, Toronto, Johannesburg

The Macmillan Publishing Company Inc.
New York

First published 1969
Second edition 1974
   Reprinted 1977, 1979

ISBN 0 7020 0521 5

*Published in the United States of America by
The Williams and Wilkins Company, Baltimore*

*Printed in Great Britain by
Billing & Sons Limited
Guildford, London and Worcester*

Preface to the Second Edition

There has been a rapid increase in the number of textbooks of pharmacology in recent years. Many of these are large, encyclopaedic, expensive and pay little attention to the specialized needs of the medical student who meets the subject at several stages during the curriculum. The purpose of this book is to provide a concise account of those aspects of pharmacology important to the medical student starting the subject and later applying it in his clinical years. The basic aspects of the subject have been emphasized throughout but no detailed practical procedures are given, as this is not possible in a book of moderate size.

There is no need to justify the teaching of basic pharmacology to the medical student. It is essential that the doctor should have a scientific and basic approach to the assessment of the drugs he uses. Pharmacology is undoubtedly the foundation of this approach, and whilst the precise drugs available or in fashion may change rapidly, their uses remain relatively constant.

In preparing the second edition considerable revision has been made throughout in an attempt to keep pace with the number of drugs becoming of recognized use since the first edition and with the increased emphasis of the importance of pharmacokinetics and pharmacodynamics. None the less, many drugs of little modern therapeutic importance are still discussed as they may represent the original classic member of their class and the standard by which the newer drugs are judged. Drugs have been grouped as far as possible under the body system which they mainly affect but the student must realize that many drugs have a variety of actions and that precise exclusive classification is not possible. Cross references must therefore be made if a comprehensive account of a particular drug is to be obtained.

This book is not intended as a therapeutic handbook and dosage of most drugs is not given. In the present era of potent drugs the precise amount to be given depends upon the individual patient and the form of dosage used. The dosage must finally be determined by the judgement and experience of the clinician concerned, but further guidance may be found in the British National Formulary, the Extra Pharmacopoeia and the manufacturers' package insert.

References are given at the end of most chapters to further reading from the standard texts or monographs on particular topics.

I am very grateful to my colleagues for their help and criticism in the revision of the book. Fig. 7 was reproduced by kind permission of the British Medical Bulletin.

May 1974   R. G. PENN

Contents

CONTENTS

CONTENTS

INTRODUCTION

Pharmacology is the study of the manner in which the functions of living organisms can be modified by chemical substances though, in the medical context, the term is usually restricted to the effects of drugs.

A drug may be defined as any substance or mixture of substances designed for administration to man for use in the diagnosis, treatment, investigation or prevention of disease or for the modification of physiological function (Committee on Safety of Drugs 1968). Many drugs are extracted from plants and include such useful substances as atropine, digitalis, and ephedrine. Some drugs, such as thyroid extract, heparin, and insulin, are extracted from animal tissue. Many of the antibiotics such as penicillin, streptomycin, and chloramphenicol were originally isolated from moulds or bacteria. Today, the most important source of drugs is chemical synthesis, and there is available a vast array of compounds of all classes and structure, some different only in minute detail. The user has to select the correct compound for his purpose and it is necessary to arrange drugs in some logical classification. It is not yet possible to do this accurately as the relationship between chemical structure and activity is known for few drugs, and most have a variety of actions which are often difficult to relate one to the other.

The mode of action of drugs at the cellular level is undergoing intensive investigation and this increased scientific understanding will undoubtedly lead to their more intelligent use.

1

Drug Names

The multiplicity of drugs gives rise to a host of names of the most confusing nature which fall into two categories as far as the therapeutic use of them is concerned.

Proprietary names. These are the registered trade marks of the firm who discovered, make or market the drug and who may have a monopoly of the manufacture. The name chosen is usually easy to remember though not always a reasonable description of the drug, as it is designed to sell and not necessarily to be informative. Other firms soon find alternatives which avoid the original patent and the result is a confusing array of drugs with different names but similar therapeutic action and chemical structure.

Approved names. A drug may be given a non-proprietary name by the British Pharmacopoeia Commission. This name will be based on a contraction of the full chemical name and is often not easy to say or remember though it will be more descriptive of the chemical class of the drug than many of the proprietary names. There is no monopoly in the use of this name so it is not popular with the drug manufacturer.

Pharmacopoeias (Gk. *pharmakon*, a drug; *-poiia*, making)

Pharmacopoeias, which are authoritative lists of drugs, their preparations, and uses, have been known since the earliest times. Today, they provide standards to guarantee the purity and activity of certain drugs which in some cases are governed by international agreement. In Great Britain the British Pharmacopoeia (B.P.) is used and amendments are made to the current edition in an Addendum which is published from time to time. The current edition of the B.P. (1973) is published by the Health Ministers on the recommendation of the Medicines Commission (see Medicines Act, page 3). Drugs recognized in the *British Pharmacopoeia* are called 'official' and have the initials B.P. placed after their name. Any method, statement or title included in the B.P. is also known as official.

The equivalent in the United States is the *United States Pharmacopeia* (U.S.P.). There is also a European Pharmacopoeia whose standards take precedence over the relevant standards of the British Pharmacopoeia.

The *British Pharmaceutical Codex* (B.P.C.) and the *Extra Pharmacopoeia* (*Martindale*), both published by the Pharmaceutical Society of Great Britain, provide much additional information on drugs which are not necessarily official. The *British National Formulary* (B.N.F.) is compiled by the Joint Formulary Committee on behalf of the Pharmaceutical Society of Great Britain and the British Medical Association. It describes the actions, uses and dosages of most of the standard preparations in current use.

Medicines Act (*1968*). Prior to this Act which came into effect in September, 1971, there was no legal requirement for any official body to approve or control the development of any new medicine on the grounds of its safety. Since the thalidomide disaster of 1962, however, the voluntary participation of doctors and the pharmaceutical industry meant that no new drugs were used without the approval of the then Dunlop Committee.

Permission to do clinical studies on any new drug or to market it must now be sought from a Licensing Authority under the direct control of the Health Ministers and Parliament. The Licensing Authority has several committees on whose advice its decisions are made. One of these, the Committee on Safety of Medicines is responsible for drugs used in human disease and has an Adverse Reactions Sub-committee which maintains a continuing surveillance of the safety of marketed drugs.

The Medicines Act also has set up a Medicines Commission to have a purely advisory function to the Licensing Authority and also to prepare and publish the British Pharmacopoeia.

To be of therapeutic use a drug must produce the required effect for the required length of time, which implies an adequate concentration of drug at the site of action.

Apart from the amount administered, there are many factors which affect the concentration or activity of a drug at the target site. These include the extent and rate of absorption; plasma or tissue binding; the rate of biotransformation and excretion; and the activity of metabolites. These processes occur simultaneously and the concentration of a drug in the body at any one time, and so the duration and intensity of its effects depend on the relative balance of these factors. The study of the absorption, distribution, metabolism and excretion of drugs is known as pharmacokinetics and the study of the biological and therapeutic effects is known as pharmacodynamics.

ABSORPTION

Save when a drug is applied for its local effect, it must reach the blood stream to be carried to the target cell. It has to pass the barriers of the skin; mucous membranes such as those lining the alimentary, respiratory and genital tracts; or if these are by-passed by injection techniques, be absorbed from subcutaneous, intramuscular and other sites. The drug will therefore have to cross a series of cell membranes which it does by diffusion, filtration through pores or by specialized transport. The latent period between the administration of the drug and the onset of effect will be determined by the route of administration, the rate of absorption, and the passage to the site of action.

The cell membrane

This is about 100 Å thick (1 Å $= 10^{-10}$ metres) and is essentially a double layer of lipid molecules sandwiched between two polypeptide layers. It has pores 4–40 Å in diameter through which hydrophilic substances may pass. The size, shape, and degree of ionization of the drug molecule and the lipid solubility of the ionized and non-ionized forms influences its passage across the cell membrane which may be by passive or active transport.

(i) *Passive transport.* Lipid soluble compounds dissolve in the membrane substance and diffuse across in proportion to the concentration gradient. The passage of a drug is favoured by a high lipid–water partition coefficient. Lipid insoluble drugs are often hydrophilic and may pass through the pores in the cell membrane if they are small enough (urea, water, small ions).

Many drugs are weak bases or acids and when in solution are present in both the ionized and non-ionized form. The ionized form is poorly soluble in lipids but the non-ionized form is usually lipid-soluble and so more easily absorbed. The equilibrium between the two forms depends upon the pK_a of the compound (the negative logarithm of the dissociation constant K_a) and the pH of the environment. When the pH equals the pK_a the drug is 50% ionized. Drugs with a low pK_a (i.e. acidic drugs) such as salicylates are mainly non-ionized in acid environments and more easily absorbed there than in an alkaline medium. The reverse is true of drugs with a high pK_a (i.e. basic drugs) such as morphine and ephedrine which are non-ionized in alkaline media. Strongly acidic or basic drugs such as streptomycin or hexamethonium will always have a large ionized fraction at the pHs found in the gut and absorption of these drugs is poor. Changes in pH may also alter the lipid-solubility of a drug; e.g. though a higher pH will lessen the non-ionized fraction of acetylsalicylic acid, it will increase the lipid solubility and the overall absorption rate may not be affected.

Similar considerations apply to drugs crossing the renal tubule cells and pH can be of considerable importance in renal excretion of drugs especially in the treatment of poisoning (page 177).

The pH gradient across the membrane will also affect the degree of ionization of the drug, and the total concentration of free drug (see also protein binding page 11) on each side of the membrane may be very different as, though the permeable non-ionized form will be in equilibrium, the amount of the ionized form (assuming it can pass the membrane) will depend on the pH and the ratio may be calculated by the Henderson–Hasselbalch equation.

(ii) *Active transport*. Some substances can cross the cell membrane against an electrical or chemical gradient, but this requires the expenditure of metabolic energy. The mechanism is probably by utilization of naturally occurring transport systems. Ions such as Na^+ and K^+, and amino acids, are carried by this method which shows selectivity, saturability and may be blocked by metabolic inhibitors. Some substances, such as glucose and the pyrimidines, are transported by a carrier mechanism but do not move against a concentration gradient. This facilitated diffusion is more rapid than simple diffusion.

Other factors influencing absorption

There are many other factors influencing absorption apart from the physicochemical properties of the cell membrane and examples will be given during the discussion of individual drugs. Drugs may be given by a variety of routes and the one used will have a major influence on the absorption and the speed and intensity of action. Routes of administration are discussed below.

Bioavailability

The active principle may be only a very small proportion of any given dose form of drug used clinically and the rest will be inert filler, buffering agents, solvents, stabilizers, etc. It has been shown quite conclusively that the biological availability (bioavailability) of the drug or the facility with which it is absorbed can be greatly influenced by the type of formulation, i.e. the other constituents of the dose form and the method of manufacture. Different formulations containing the same amount of active drug can therefore lead to marked differences in clinical effectiveness. This was strikingly shown recently when lactose was substituted for calcium sulphate as a filler in phenytoin capsules and led to a marked rise in absorption and consequent toxicity. Different formulations of 0·5 mg digoxin have also been shown recently to give a seven fold difference in peak plasma levels. It should be noted that adherence to present British Pharmacopoeial standards does not ensure similar bioavailability between formulations as this is not officially required to be measured.

Absorption of the active drug from a tablet or a capsule is preceded by disintegration of the vehicle, dispersion of the drug particles and their dissolution in the gastrointestinal fluid. Manufacturing processes can change the rate of disintegration and as it is the dissolved drug which is absorbed, the longer this takes or the more insoluble the drug, the longer it will take to be absorbed. The particle size will also have an influence as the smaller the particle, the larger its surface area in proportion to its size and hence it will dissolve more rapidly. These factors are made use of in delay preparations which have prolonged absorption times and hence have more prolonged blood levels than a more soluble form of the drug.

The rate of absorption will also be influenced by the circulation to the site of administration. If this is large then absorption will be fast; hence drugs which are vasoconstrictors will delay absorption which will also be slow from areas with a poor supply (such as the subcutaneous tissue in surgical shock).

ROUTES OF ADMINISTRATION

1. Oral administration

This route has the advantages of being easy with no need for a sterile preparation. Absorption takes place mainly in the intestine though some substances, such as alcohol, are partly absorbed from the gastric mucosa. The activity and contents of the stomach may therefore be important factors. Irritant drugs may cause spasm of the pylorus or even vomiting.

Water-soluble compounds of small molecular weight, such as urea, are rapidly and passively absorbed, though larger molecules may need an active transport system. The effect of pH and lipid solubility on absorption has already been discussed (page 5).

Drugs may not be effective by the oral route for several reasons. Absorption of streptomycin and neomycin may be so poor as to be negligible. Some drugs are destroyed in the gut lumen; insulin, corticotrophin and vasopressin are destroyed by enzyme action, benzylpenicillin is destroyed by stomach acid and histamine is destroyed by bacterial action. Some drugs may be absorbed from the gut but are so rapidly destroyed in the liver as to be therapeutically ineffective. These drugs, such as glyceryl trinitrate, may sometimes be given satisfactorily by the sublingual route (page 9). The absorption of certain drugs may be influenced by unsatisfactory pharmaceutical formulation (see bioavailability page 6) and in extreme cases, as with some enteric coated preparations, the drug may pass through the bowel unabsorbed.

2. Parenteral administration (Gk. *para*, beside; *enteron*, intestine)

This is usually taken to mean 'by injection', though strictly could be applied to any route other than the gut. Parenteral administration is sometimes essential for the drug to be absorbed in an active form; for a speedy action; or if the patient is unable to take drugs by mouth. Drugs given by injection must be sterile and a certain amount of skill is necessary.

(i) *Intradermal injection.* Here a minute amount of drug is placed in the skin where it may remain localized for some time. This method is used in various diagnostic tests such as the Mantoux test or in the administration of some vaccines such as BCG.

(ii) *Subcutaneous (hypodermic) injection.* Here absorption is slow and even and depends on the local blood flow and the area over which the drug is spread. It is slowed by vasoconstriction or by implanting a pellet of the drug under the skin (as absorption is proportional to the surface area of the drug). Absorption may be speeded up by the concurrent use of such drugs as hyaluronidase which breaks down intercellular connections and allows the drug to spread and have a larger area for absorption. Irritant drugs should not be given subcutaneously as they cause pain and maybe necrosis of the skin.

(iii) *Intramuscular injection.* Irritant drugs such as streptomycin, mersalyl and paraldehyde can be given by this route, but necrosis can still occur. Absorption is more rapid than by subcutaneous injection but is subject to similar influences.

(iv) *Intravenous injection.* Here there is no trouble about absorption as the drug is put straight into the blood stream and irritant drugs can be given this way as they are rapidly diluted though thrombosis and thrombophlebitis can occur. As the normal blocks to absorption are absent, the onset of action of the drug will be very rapid, though not immediate, and it may take two or three circulation times for full mixing and effects to occur.

The effects could easily reach dangerous levels with drugs like adrenaline, where the influence of the injection 'slug' on the heart before full mixing occurs could easily provoke severe toxic reactions.

(v) *Other parenteral sites.* There are other less usual sites of parenteral administration. Drugs may be given via the bone marrow in babies or older patients where veins cannot be entered, as the effect is very similar to intravenous injection. Administration of drugs into the subarachnoid space (intrathecal injection) is used to circumvent the blood–brain barrier when antibiotics are being given for central nervous infections or when local anaesthetics are used in spinal anaesthesia. Local anaesthetics may also be injected into the epidural space. Intra-arterial injection gives intense localized effects and radio-opaque material may be injected by this route to make the arteries visible on X-ray (arteriography). Drugs may also be given intra-arterially for the localized treatment of cancer.

3. Application to mucous membranes

Drugs are usually applied to mucous membranes for their local or topical effect, though absorption can sometimes be very rapid and practically equivalent to intravenous administration.

(i) *Sublingual mucosa.* Drugs such as glyceryl trinitrate are rapidly destroyed in the liver if absorbed via the hepatic portal system but, if dissolved under the tongue, they rapidly and completely pass into the systemic system. The sublingual route is an efficient method though not suitable for irritant or unpleasant tasting drugs.

(ii) *Rectal mucosa.* This is often of use if the oral route cannot be used because of vomiting or in an unconscious patient. Absorption is often irregular and incomplete though water, salts and simple sugars can be given satisfactorily.

(iii) *Other mucosae.* The mucosae of other areas such as the vagina, urethra, conjunctiva, nose and nasopharynx often have drugs applied to them for topical use, though in some cases, as when using local anaesthetics, absorption may be sufficient to give systemic toxic effects. Drugs such as cocaine or pituitary snuff may be inhaled or blown into the nose.

4. The pulmonary epithelium

This method has its major application in the inhalation of volatile and gaseous anaesthetics and is discussed on page 214. Some drugs may be given as metered doses of aerosols or powder for local effect. Isoprenaline, for example, is used for its broncho-dilating action to terminate asthmatic attacks.

5. The skin

Very few drugs penetrate the intact skin and their absorption depends on their lipid solubility. Drugs may be rubbed into the skin (inunction) or driven into the skin by a galvanic current (iontophoresis). Drugs may be absorbed from a damaged or inflamed skin.

DISTRIBUTION

The body may be considered as a series of linked compartments of differing accessibility to a drug dependent on such factors as its lipid solubility, pK_a, binding to plasma protein.

1. *The body compartments.* Once in the blood stream, distribution of a drug around the body is usually very rapid but complete equilibrium may take some time in areas like the bone marrow and adipose tissue which are poorly supplied with blood. Most drugs eventually distribute throughout the total body water (75% of the body weight, or 50 litres), though this may be slow and incomplete. Drugs such as urea, alcohol, salicylates and sulphonamides are fairly rapidly distributed throughout the total body water. Certain drugs such as some dyes are practically limited to the plasma volume (3 litres) as they are very protein bound. Other drugs such as iodides, thiocyanates, inorganic bromides and quaternary compounds are virtually restricted to the extracellular space (about 25% of the total body weight). Some drugs such as streptomycin and penicillin may not easily pass the blood–brain barrier to enter the cerebrospinal fluid and it may be necessary to give them intrathecally if action on the CNS is wanted.

2. *Preferential accumulation.* Some drugs have preferential sites of accumulation in particular tissues. Various dyes and the antimalarial drug mepacrine are concentrated in cells many times that of the plasma, probably in relation to the nuclear material. The body fat, which even in a lean person is some 20% of the body weight, has a high affinity for some drugs such as thiopentone and ether. This binding by the fat depots is a very potent method of terminating the action of such drugs, but will lessen with repeated doses as the depots become saturated. The thyroid, salivary glands, and the gastric mucosa selectively concentrate iodide, thiocyanate, perchlorate and nitrate which each competitively interfere with the uptake of the others. Lead is characteristically sequestered in bone and soon cumulates to give toxic effects. Sometimes the organs of excretion such as the kidney and the liver have a higher concentration of drug than the organ upon which the drug predominantly acts.

3. *Binding to plasma protein.* Many drugs are bound to protein in the plasma, especially the albumin fraction. This decreases their biotransformation and renal excretion, and prolongs their action. It also limits the therapeutically effective blood concentration as only the unbound drug is active. Some drugs such as thyroxine, hydrocortisone, phenylbutazone and the long acting sulphonamides are nearly completely bound. The figure for the plasma level of a drug has therefore a very limited meaning unless protein binding is taken into account.

Some drugs may compete for the same site on the plasma proteins and displace a drug already there. This may have great practical importance for as it is the non-bound (free) fraction which is pharmacologically active, even small displacements of highly bound drugs can cause the free drug level to rise into the toxic range. For example, if a patient is stabilized on the anticoagulant warfarin but then takes salicylates, these may displace some of the highly protein bound warfarin to increase the anticoagulant effect and so cause bleeding.

The degree of binding is also influenced by the concentration of plasma proteins. Customary dosage schedules of a drug (which take into account normal protein binding) may therefore be upset in hypoproteinaemic states or in pregnancy (where there is a rise in plasma protein).

4. *Placental transfer.* Drugs can pass across the placental

membranes especially non-ionized drugs of high fat solubility. They may produce toxic effects in the fetus or induce congenital abnormalities (page 34).

5. *The brain*. The same general principles derived from the lipid solubility, pK$_a$ and protein binding of a drug apply to its passage into the brain (the blood–brain barrier). If a substance does not easily pass into the brain, it is sometimes possible to give a precursor which will do so. (See levodopa, page 52.)

BIOTRANSFORMATION OF DRUGS

Detoxication

This is the metabolism by the body of compounds not normally found in it, but the term is a bad one as some drugs become more active or toxic. Many drugs are lipid soluble or weak electrolytes and easily reabsorbed by the renal tubules, so to be excreted, they must be changed to more ionized and less lipid-soluble compounds. These changes may be by non-synthetic reactions such as oxidations, reductions, hydrolyses, which introduce or unmask functional groups for a second and synthetic phase in which the drug or its metabolites is conjugated with endogenous molecules such as glucuronic acid, sulphates, acetyl groups, methyl groups or amino acids. This masks the active groups, makes the compound more polar and less lipid soluble, and so facilitates excretion. These reactions occur mainly in the liver but also in the plasma, kidneys, intestinal mucosa and other tissues.

Microsomal drug metabolizing enzymes. Although some compounds may be inactivated by the enzymes involved in intermediary metabolism, biotransformation occurs especially by the microsomal drug metabolizing enzymes of the liver. These are found in the endoplasmic reticulum of the cell which on homogenization and differential centrifugation separates as the ribosome containing rough endoplasmic reticulum (ER) and the smooth endoplasmic reticulum (SER). The SER has no ribosomes but breaks into fragments called microsomes which contain the enzymes.

Obviously there cannot be in advance a specific microsomal system for every possible compound that enters the body and the number of metabolic pathways by which drugs can be handled is limited and the enzymes are non-specific acting on molecular groups rather than particular compounds. Sometimes the concurrent administration of several drugs causes competition for these pathways. Some compounds, such as SKF 525 A, will inhibit the microsomal enzymes and so prolong the action of drugs like hexobarbitone, though this inhibition may be succeeded by stimulation. Similarly, if the liver is damaged or in immature babies where the enzymes are deficient, the metabolism of drugs such as pethidine, morphine, and chloramphenicol can be greatly prolonged.

Some drugs are metabolized at sites other than the microsomal system such as the cytoplasm, mitochondria and the plasma. Other drugs also undergo change in the gut due to the action of the intestinal microflora. This may be of importance in those drugs which are excreted via the bile and absorbed again in the gut (the enterohepatic circulation).

Enzyme induction. Continued administration of some drugs stimulates the formation of microsomal enzymes (enzyme induction). Significant enzyme induction generally occurs after a few days administration of the inducing drug and ceases within several weeks after the drug administration is stopped. Such drugs will therefore enhance their own rate of metabolism and, owing to the non-specificity of the microsomal enzymes, the metabolism of other drugs and even normal constituents of the body may be affected. An increasing number of drugs are known to induce enzymes in this manner and include phenylbutazone, phenobarbitone, meprobamate, caffeine and ethanol. Enzyme induction can cause tolerance to a drug (page 23) and account for some drug–drug interactions (page 38).

The metabolism of drugs *in vivo*

Some drugs are excreted largely unchanged. Examples are barbitone, which is highly polar and does not easily penetrate the cell, and ether which is very volatile and quickly passes out via the lungs. Most drugs are metabolized by routes which may be exceedingly complex and follow many different paths of metabolic transformation, and the number of different metabolites of some drugs exceeds a hundred or more. Individual examples of these changes are:

(i) *Oxidations.* These occur especially in the liver microsomes and may involve dehydrogenation, hydroxylation, dealkylation and deamination. Examples are the oxidation of ethanol by alcohol dehydrogenase to acetaldehyde (and further to acetate and then carbon dioxide and water) and the oxidative deamination of noradrenaline by monoamine oxidase.

(ii) *Reductions.* Chloral hydrate is reduced to trichloroethanol.

(iii) *Hydrolyses.* Many esters and amides are hydrolysed. Acetylcholine is de-esterified to choline and acetate. Local anaesthetics such as procaine are hydrolysed to p-aminobenzoic acid and diethylaminoethanol.

(iv) *Conjugations.* After biotransformation to salicylic acid, acetylsalicylic acid is conjugated with glycine to form salicyluric acid.

Further examples of biotransformations are given when dealing with the individual drugs. Sometimes it is the metabolic product which is the active principle; e.g. chloral hydrate is reduced to the active trichloroethanol; phenacetin which has some action of its own is oxidized to the more active paracetamol; *in vivo* cyclization of the antimalarial drug paludrine to give the active compound.

Factors Affecting the Metabolism of a Drug

The metabolism of a drug is influenced by many factors which account in large part for the individual and species differences of the response (see Chapter 4). These factors are genetic, physiological, pharmacodynamic and environmental.

1. *Genetic factors.* There is often great species difference in the handling of a drug and the qualitative and quantitative response to it. Whilst the basic metabolic transformations such as oxidation, reduction and hydrolysis are fairly similar in most species, conjugation mechanisms often have characteristic differences which show some degree of phylogenetic development.

There may also be variations in the pattern of metabolism of drugs in the same species. A classic example is due to a genetically determined deficiency of glucose-6-phosphate dehydrogenase in the red blood cell when drugs such as primaquine, pamaquine and p-aminosalicylic acid cause an oxidative denaturation of haemoglobin and haemolysis. This enzyme deficiency occurs characteristically in Negroes, non-Ashkenazi Jews and Sardinians and has the peculiar property of being associated with an inherited resistance to *P. falciparum* malaria.

Other examples of genetically determined abnormalities in drug handling are isoniazid (page 267) and in deficiency of plasma pseudocholinesterase (page 83).

2. *Physiological factors.* Age may have a pronounced effect on the handling of drugs. The fetal and newborn animal has a limited capacity to metabolize drugs such as chloramphenicol due to the immaturity of the liver microsomal system, which in the human is not fully developed till eight weeks of age. This may result in prolonged activity and increased toxicity of many drugs. Liver disease can have a similar effect. Hormones may also alter drug handling, and pregnancy or the use of sex hormones (e.g. oral contraception) can result in changes of protein binding.

The activity of many drug metabolizing enzymes is also dependent on the nutritional status of the animal and deficiencies of protein, minerals, ascorbic acid and other vitamins may have marked effects.

3. *Pharmacodynamic and environmental factors.* The metabolism of a drug is very dependent on tissue distribution, plasma protein binding and competition with other drugs, endogenous compounds, food additives and pesticide residues occurring in the diet. These factors are discussed elsewhere in this chapter.

EXCRETION

The elimination of drugs and metabolites from the body is mainly via the kidneys, though the lungs are important for the removal of volatile and gaseous general anaesthetics and for about one-fifth of administered paraldehyde. Some drugs are excreted in saliva (heavy metals), sweat (paraldehyde), tears, gastric and bronchial gland secretion, in the colon and across the placenta. Some products of metabolism may be excreted in the bile and be reabsorbed in the intestine (e.g. phenolphthalein). This enterohepatic circulation is of importance in the prolongation of action of some drugs. Excretion via the milk may affect the suckling infant.

The mechanisms of renal excretion are passive filtration at the glomerulus, tubular secretion and reabsorption. The free drug is filtered at the glomerulus so protein binding will reduce the amount available for this. Once in the tubules, the non-ionized form is readily reabsorbed (cf. the gut epithelium) and hence excretion will be low. The ionized form is poorly reabsorbed and so excreted. By increasing the formation of urine with diuretics and decreasing the reabsorption of the drug by appropriate change of urinary pH (page 177) maximal excretion of a drug occurs. This forced diuresis is used in the treatment of some acute poisoning, e.g. with phenobarbitone.

The alteration of excretion rate which is caused by a change in urinary pH may also upset the expected dose–effect relationship. Mecamylamine, for example, is predominantly non-ionized in alkaline urine and is reabsorbed thus potentiating the effect of a single dose.

Some compounds such as penicillin are actively secreted via the kidney tubules and this can be blocked by drugs such as probenecid.

Rate of clearance of drugs

The process or removal of a drug from the body is known as clearance and the great majority of drugs are cleared in an exponential fashion, that is the amount removed in unit time is a constant fraction of the amount still present. The rate of clearance may be conveniently expressed as the *plasma half-life* $(T_{\frac{1}{2}})$ i.e. the time taken for the plasma concentration to fall to a half though the *biological half-life* is often used and is the time taken for the total amount of drug in the body (not necessarily the same as the plasma concentration e.g. where there is uneven distribution) to fall to half. It must also be remembered that whereas the plasma concentration (and hence the plasma half-life) usually gives a measure of the duration and magnitude of effect, this is not always so. Some drugs, e.g. vitamin D, are rapidly cleared from the plasma but stored in the tissues. Some drugs, e.g. monoamine oxidase inhibitors, reserpine, have effects which last after the disappearance of the drug from the plasma ('hit and run').

Plasma half-lives vary markedly from drug to drug and some drugs such as benzylpenicillin, tubocurarine are so rapidly cleared that this is a major factor in the limitation of the intensity and duration of their action and half clearance may occur in less than half an hour. Most drugs have a half-life of 4–24 hours though some such as digoxin, thyroxine and arsenic are cleared extremely slowly and half-clearance takes days.

Frequency of administration

In therapeutic use an effective level of drug must be maintained at the site of action for the appropriate time. Obviously the amount administered must take into account the rapidity with which the drug is cleared from the body.

As the relationship of plasma concentration and time is usually exponential it follows that a single dose of a drug would have to be increased markedly to double the duration of action, i.e. the relationship between dose and duration of action is NOT linear. Increasing the dose this way could easily cause toxic levels to be reached in the early stages of absorption and so drugs are often given, not as single doses, but as a series of doses whose size and interval is calculated to maintain the optimum blood levels.

Accumulation. If a drug is administered over a period of time, it is possible to give it at a faster rate than it is excreted. The body level of the drug will rise until the amount cleared in the interval between doses is equal to a single dose. If a drug is given at intervals corresponding to its half-life, the plasma concentration will rise to a steady state in about 4 half-lives at which time the concentration will fluctuate between the maximum concentration produced by the first dose and twice that level. If a dose is calculated to maintain the therapeutic plasma level, this will therefore not be reached for some little time and so large initial doses are often given (loading doses) till the required blood level is reached and this therapeutic level is then maintained by smaller doses (maintenance doses) which just balance clearance.

Toxic levels can easily be reached especially with drugs which are cleared slowly such as thyroxine and digoxin.

Calculation of dose

A drug has no standard dose which works equally well in every patient regardless of age, sex, weight and other individual variables as should be clear from the discussion on pharmacological variation (page 28). With many drugs the effective dose is well below the toxic level so a fixed amount may be used which is enough to make individual variation unimportant. Sometimes it is necessary to calculate the dose more exactly. This is often done on a mg drug/kg body weight basis though a dose based on body surface area or blood volume might be better. Dosage of a drug may also be carefully adjusted over a period according to the response desired as with antihypertensives, insulins, anticoagulants, general anaesthetics, etc.

It must always be remembered that a drug is given to an individual who may not be typical of the population at large. Various factors may influence the individual response and are considered elsewhere in this book. It is essential in these days of potent drugs, often with a narrow margin between therapeutic effect and toxicity, to study the appropriate literature, both official compendia and manufacturers' package inserts, and to calculate the dose on scientific principles not guess-work.

REFERENCES

Aldridge, W. N. (ed.) (1969) Mechanisms of toxicity. *Brit. med. Bull.*, **25**, 3.

Barlow, R. B. (1964) *Introduction to Chemical Pharmacology*, 2nd edn. London: Methuen.

Binns, T. B. (ed.) (1964) *Absorption and Distribution of Drugs.* Edinburgh: Livingstone.

Northcote, D. H. (ed.) (1968) Structure and function of membranes. *Brit. med. Bull.*, **24**, 2.

La Du, B. N., Mandel, H. G. & Way, E. L. (eds.) (1971) *Fundamentals of Drug Metabolism and Drug Disposition.* Edinburgh and London: Churchill Livingstone.

Parke, D. V. (1968) Metabolism of drugs and factors which affect the metabolism of drugs. In *Recent Advances in Pharmacology*, 4th edn. Robson, J. M. & Stacey, R. S. (eds.). pp. 29–98. London: Churchill.

BASIC MECHANISMS OF DRUG ACTION

It is important to realize that drugs can only increase or decrease established functions of the cell such as excitability, contractibility, rhythmicity and secretion and cannot impart new functions. That is, drugs can change the action of a cell quantitatively and only by stimulation or depression. The cell is essentially a pool of enzymes bounded by a membrane and has energy-using and energy-producing reactions. A drug may act on any of these sites and what is known of the mechanisms of action and their relationship to chemical structure will be discussed with the individual drugs.

1. The drug receptor

Obvious effects may be produced on the eserinized leech with acetylcholine in dilutions of one in a thousand million. The ordinary chemical laws are still obeyed for, even at these dilutions, there are still vast numbers of interacting molecular groups. Drugs often have great selectivity in the cells they influence and may affect a single type only. It is obvious that the drug must work at a special site in the cell as it is not in sufficient concentration to cover more than a very small percentage of the cell surface. Sometimes this specialized site can be anatomically demonstrated as, for example, the motor end plate. These factors give rise to the concept of the 'drug receptor' which is thought to be a specialized area of the cell surface with which drugs react to produce their

19

effect. The cell is a complex, organized and correlated system of enzymes, and it is not surprising that interference at only one site could bring about marked biochemical and physiological change.

Langley by 1878 had coined the phrase 'receptive substance' and suggested that the drug–cell combination obeyed the Law of Mass Action. Conceived by Ehrlich to be like a piece of mosaic finding its place in a pattern, the drug-receptor complex is now thought of as a spatially organized chemical interaction whereby only a drug with the appropriately arranged chemical groups is able to react in a complementary fashion with the cell surface. This reaction mainly involves ionic and other relatively weak and reversible bonds, though sometimes firmer covalent bonds are concerned. The selectivity of drugs depends on these spatially organized chemical interactions for even slight changes of the three-dimensional structure may prevent the close apposition of drug and receptor and the triggering of the usual response (steric hindrance). A characteristic property of receptors is this specificity and each drug acts on a particular type of receptor. Sometimes different drugs may act on the same receptors, as, for example, adrenaline and noradrenaline, though drugs may act on different receptors and produce the same apparent effect (e.g. cocaine and atropine both produce dilatation of the pupil). Identity of receptors may be shown by the use of competitive antagonists (page 22).

Many attempts have been made to describe mathematically the drug–receptor relationship and the effects of combinations of drugs which act on the same receptor. The classical theory of Clark said that the drug effect was proportional to the fraction of receptors occupied and that maximum effect occurred when none were left vacant, though later theories assume that maximum effect is possible even if some receptors are not occupied (spare receptors).

The tendency of a drug to combine with the receptor (the affinity) may be separated from the tendency of the drug–receptor complex to elicit a response (intrinsic activity or efficacy). A drug which has both affinity and efficacy (the agonist) will produce a response, whereas a drug which has affinity but no efficacy (an antagonist) will not elicit a response and may hinder an agonist from doing so. A partial agonist has affinity but less intrinsic activity than the full agonist on the same receptor and summation of effect or antagonism may occur depending on the drugs and their relative concentrations.

According to Paton, however, the excitation of a receptor is due to the rate of combination and not merely the occupancy of a receptor. He states that if the drug–receptor complex can dissociate rapidly and so leave the receptor free for further combination and so on, then the action of the drug will be stimulant as each formation of the drug–receptor complex gives, as it were, a quantum of action. If, however, the drug–receptor complex is firmly bound and unable to dissociate then no further stimulation can occur and the effect will be antagonistic. As even antagonists at first must combine with and excite the receptor, an initial stimulant effect is sometimes seen. The firmness of the drug–receptor complex explains why it is often so difficult to wash out antagonists and why they may take some time to develop their action.

At the present time it is not possible to choose between the various receptor theories but they provide a useful conceptual framework.

2. Non-specific mechanisms

It is usual to refer to the term 'drug receptor' only when the drug–cell combination initiates obvious effects. Some drugs, however, seem less specific and do not interact with receptors. They may, for instance, bind to plasma protein or to enzymes concerned in metabolism, biotransformation or transport. Drugs may also act by virtue of their physical properties such as solubility in fat which allows of accumulation in the lipid phase of the cell, e.g. the volatile anaesthetics. Some drugs may also act by direct chemical interactions, e.g. antacids and chelating agents.

COMBINATIONS OF DRUGS

If two or more drugs are given at the same time, their effects may interact in various ways.

Antagonism

If the effect of a drug is decreased or abolished by another, this is termed antagonism. It may be of several sorts:

(i) *Physiological* (*non-competitive*) *antagonism.* This occurs when two drugs act on different receptors and have opposite physical effects. An example is the action of histamine and adrenaline on the bronchial muscle.

(ii) *Chemical antagonism.* This occurs when the antagonist combines with the agonist to form an inactive complex. An example is dimercaprol and mercury (page 171).

(iii) *Unsurmountable antagonism.* This is due to an irreversible inactivation of the receptor site, as, for example, dibenamine and the α-adrenergic receptor.

(iv) *Competitive antagonism* (*substrate competition*). If the agonist and the antagonist act reversibly at the same receptor, the interaction may be described by a simple mathematical relationship if it is assumed that the agonist and the antagonist compete for the receptor according to the Law of Mass Action. This means that if the presence of the antagonist reduces the effect of the agonist then the original response can be obtained by increasing the concentration of the agonist. In competitive antagonism, if the log-dose response curves of the agonist are plotted for different concentrations of antagonist; these lines will be parallel (Fig. 1). If two agonists act on the same receptor they will be similarly antagonized by the same competitive antagonist, and all similar receptors will have the same affinity for the same agonist. This permits receptors to be identified.

Examples of competitive antagonism are curare and acetylcholine (page 81), morphine and nalorphine (page 184), sulphonamides and ρ-aminobenzoic acid (page 260), histamine and the competitive antihistamines (page 89).

Synergism (Gk. *sun* together; *ergos*, work)

This is said to occur when two drugs act in the same way together. If the total effect is the simple arithmetic sum of the individual effects, this is said to be addition. If the magnitude of the effects of a drug mixture is greater than the sum of the individual effects of the component drugs, this is said to be potentiation. There is, however, some equivocation over the meaning of these words and for some, synergism is the same as potentiation and for others potentiation means sensitization.

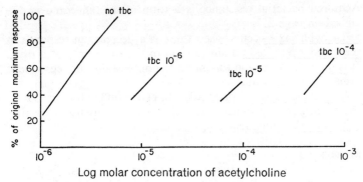

FIG. 1. Competitive antagonism. This figure shows the parallel log-dose response curves characteristic of competitive antagonism.

The frog rectus abdominis contracts when acetylcholine (the agonist) is added to it, but in the presence of the antagonist tubocurarine (tbc), increased amounts of acetylcholine are needed to restore the original response. (Taken from a class experiment.)

Drug–drug interactions ('pharmacokinetic drug interactions')

Although many drug interactions are desired and are discussed under the relevant headings, some of them are the cause of unexpected adverse reactions in the therapeutic use of drugs (see page 36).

Tolerance and tachyphylaxis (Gk. *takhus*, swift; *phulaxis*, a guarding)

Tolerance occurs when there is a decrease in response to the repeated administration of a drug. It is slow in onset and the original effect is produced by increasing the dose. The mechanisms and types of tolerance are various. It can be acquired perhaps due to decrease of sensitivity of receptor sites or enzyme induction (page 13). A classical example of acquired tolerance is to opiates by the drug abuser (see page 237). Certain types of tolerance (natural, species) are due to genetically determined causes, often an increased metabolism of the drug. Cross tolerance can also occur to other drugs not always of the same chemical class.

Acquired bacterial resistance is a form of tolerance and is discussed on page 257.

Tachyphylaxis occurs when there is a decrease in response to the rapidly repeated administration of the same dose of a drug. It is quick in onset and the initial response cannot be reproduced even with a larger dose.

It is difficult to be dogmatic about the individual causes of these various phenomena, and they will be discussed as they arise with the individual drugs.

REFERENCES

Van Rossum, J. M. (1968) Drug receptor theories. In *Recent Advances in Pharmacology*, 4th edn. Robson, J. M. & Stacey, R. S. (eds.). pp. 99–134. London: Churchill.

Waud, D. R. (1968) Pharmacological receptors. *Pharmacological Reviews*, **20**, 49.

It is customary to describe the effects of drugs in terms of biochemical, physiological or symptomatic change and to express these changes in quantitative terms related to such parameters as dosage, variability, selectivity, intensity and time course of effect.

DOSE–RESPONSE CURVES

The magnitude of a selected drug effect is a function of the dose given or, more precisely, the molar concentration presented to the effector cell, and it is possible to describe the relationship between dose and response by a curve whose shape depends on the biological object, the response measured, and the drug employed, and there is a characteristic curve for specified sets of conditions. It is customary to plot the dose on the abscissa (horizontal scale) and the response on the ordinate (vertical scale).

The intensity of the drug effect is commonly taken to be the peak effect of a single dose or the average effect of chronic dosage so its magnitude is a function of time as well as dose. There are two basic forms of dose–response curve.

1. *Graded (quantitative) dose–response curves.* Here the dose of the drug is related to the degree of response in a single biological unit and the amount of response in each unit is proportional to the amount of drug. The response to a particular dose is measured in absolute units or as a percentage of the maximum possible response. A typical example is the action of histamine on the contraction of the longitudinal muscle of the guinea-pig ileum. The response increases in a gradual fashion with increasing

25

amounts of drug once a threshold concentration is reached and rises to a ceiling or maximum level. The type of curve is characteristic for the particular kind of conditions. It is generally convex upwards if plotted on an arithmetic scale (Fig. 2) but if the dose

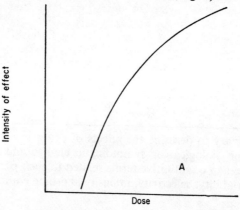

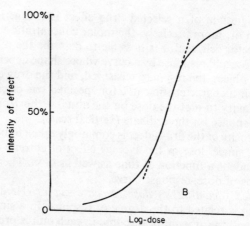

FIG. 2. Graded dose–response curves.

(A) The graded dose–response curve may be plotted as the relationship between the effect and the dose. This relationship is usually hyperbolic.

(B) It may also be plotted as the relationship between the effect, usually as a percentage of the maximum effect, and the logarithm of the dose. This relationship is almost linear in the middle range.

is plotted logarithmically, the convexity diminishes and the line becomes approximately straight over the central part of the curve (between about 25 and 75% of the maximal response). The linear part cannot be extrapolated far for obviously the effect does not increase indefinitely with dose and, at the other end of the line, negative results do not occur with a less than threshold dose. In many cases, especially on isolated organs, the log dose–response curve is sigmoid. The reason for this is not known but is mathematically descriptive of a reversible combination of drug and tissue governed by the Mass Action Laws, as for example also occurs in the titration curve of a buffer or in the oxyhaemoglobin dissociation curve.

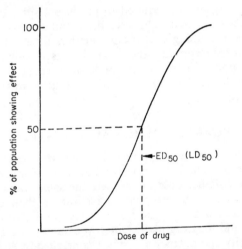

FIG. 3. Quantal dose–response curves. This type of curve demonstrates the relationship between the dose of a drug and the proportion of a population showing a given effect. It is used especially in the determination of the acute toxicity of a drug by recording the percentage of a group affected by increase of dose. The dose causing 50% of the population to be affected is the median effective dose or the ED50 (or the LD50 if the effect measured is death).

2. *Quantal (all or none) dose–response curves.* This type of curve demonstrates the relationship between the dose of a drug and the proportion of a population of biological units showing the given effect. Each unit responds maximally but the number

of units responding depends on the drug concentration. This relationship is seen in determinations of the acute toxicity of a drug by recording the percentage of a group affected by increasing dose (see page 34). Quite often the curve is of a gaussian or normal distribution (Fig. 3) but sometimes there may be extraneous effects in some dose ranges which modify the curve. It is possible to use other graphic forms for the analysis of quantal dose–response data such as the Normal Equivalent Deviation (NED) and the Probit. A textbook of statistics should be consulted for details.

Potency and efficacy

The absolute weights required to produce a specific effect are used to make comparisons between drugs (relative potency). This can be very misleading as it usually matters little if 1 μg of one drug is required to produce the same effect as 100 mg of another. What is important is maximum or 'ceiling' effect possible with each drug (relative efficacy) and if this is restricted by the presence of side effects.

PHARMACOLOGICAL VARIATION

A dose–response curve applies only to a particular individual or the average individual of a group and another individual may not respond to a similar dose in precisely the same way though this variation is likely to be quantitative rather than qualitative. Variation in pharmacological response has two major causes; the individual and the drug itself. Different samples of the drug may vary in purity and potency and this is controlled by standardizing its manufacture, storage and distribution (see Biological Standardization, page 30).

Individual Variation

If the same dose of drug is given to a group of subjects, there is a range of intensity of effects and similarly there is a range of doses required to produce a standard effect, and variation may be expressed in either of these ways. The variation may be somewhat unevenly distributed through the population and give a skew curve rather than the typical bell-shaped normal curve (figure 4), though this may often be converted to a symmetrical distribution if the doses are plotted logarithmically. The amount of scatter depends on the particular population and may be less in inbred populations. Some drugs such as digitalis and the general anaesthetics have a narrow scatter.

The data may also be plotted as an Integrated Frequency Distribution Curve to show the percentage of subjects responding to a given dose (Fig. 4). This allows measurement of the median effective dose (ED50) or that dose which affects 50% of a population. By using other parameters such as logarithmic and probability scales, the sigmoid curve may be made linear which facilitates statistical analysis.

Even the same individual may not respond similarly to the same drug on different occasions owing to a constantly changing physiological and biochemical milieu especially if this has been modified by the presence of other drugs or pathological factors.

Many factors influence the variation of the response in different individuals (see also page 14). It has been said already that the effect of a drug is related to the molar concentration at the effector cell. The same standard dose will produce different effective concentrations in subjects of different body weight and so dose and effect should always be related to body weight (and perhaps also to body surface area or to blood volume). Women are supposedly different from men in some of their reactions to drugs, though the effect of a standard dosage schedule in the (usually) lighter female may be of importance.

Age influences the response to some drugs and young children are especially sensitive to drugs which depress the central nervous system. Immature babies are unable to metabolize some drugs properly (see page 15), and in the older person there is increased likelihood of other pathology modifying the ability to inactivate and excrete drugs though this can be a factor at any age.

Although all pharmacological responses are affected by hereditary factors, the responses of some individuals to certain drugs may be very unusual (see Idiosyncrasy, page 37). Other factors to be considered include the concurrent or prior administration of other drugs; the route by which the drug is given and its absorption, distribution and biotransformation (Chapter 2).

Different species may respond entirely differently and it is not possible to extrapolate dose–effect in one species to that in another without a great deal of ancillary comparison and experience. The marked species variability in response to a given dose of a drug was previously attributed to intrinsic differences in the responsiveness of the target organ based on the assumption that the same dose of drug (mg/kg) attained the same concentration at the drug receptors in the different species. This does not appear to be the complete answer, however, and variations in response seem to be also dependent on different metabolic handling producing differences in the amount of drug reaching the site of action. Both inter and intraspecies response seem to be much more correlated with the plasma concentration than to the absolute dosage.

Biological Standardization

In order to administer them satisfactorily, the potency of drugs must be known and conform to a standard of uniform activity from one batch of manufacture to the next. This is normally done by chemical or physical methods, but where this is not possible (if, for example, there is no reliable or sensitive enough method) then living organisms or tissue must be used.

Biological assay

This is the determination of the potency of a physical, chemical or biological agent by means of a biological indicator; that is, by its effect on living animals or tissue. Although biological responses are so variable, it is possible to get almost any required degree of accuracy by repeating the tests and analysing them statistically to find not only the activity of the test preparation but the limits of error of the assay. Biological assay is not required for the majority of drugs though it is still used for some hormones and vitamins and a few miscellaneous drugs such as digitalis. Biological assay is also used in research and in diagnosis to detect very small amounts of physiologically active substances if this cannot be done by other means.

Normally, a sample and a standard preparation are compared and there may be qualitative or quantitative difference between them. Methods where there are qualitative differences between the two preparations are used to compare the activity of a new drug

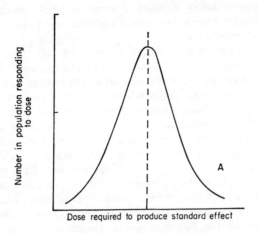

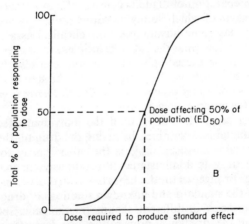

FIG. 4. Individual variation in response to drugs.

Graph (A) shows the relationship between the dose of a drug required to produce a standard effect and the number in a population responding to that dose. This frequency distribution curve is usually bell shaped.

Graph (B): the same data may be plotted as an integrated frequency curve by showing the total percentage of the population responding to a given dose. This allows measurement of the ED50 or that dose which affects 50% of the population.

with that of another; for example, a new analgesic with morphine (comparative or screening assay). The results depend on the method and the species and can give only a preliminary indication of the relative activity in man.

If there is merely a quantitative difference between the sample and the standard, and each contains different amounts of the same drug, the final result does not depend on the method or the species and the response does not have to be the same as the therapeutic use of the drug. This is the type of assay used to standardize drugs (analytical or dilution assay). In many cases an International Standard Preparation is available and this or standards derived from it are used in the assay of the unknown sample. The potency of the sample is measured in units where a unit of the given drug is the amount of specific activity contained in an arbitrarily fixed weight of the respective stable standard preparation. The methods of preparing the standard and of performing the assay are precisely defined for Pharmacopoeial preparations, e.g. the B.P. standard preparation of digitalis consists of a mixture of *Digitalis purpurea* leaves of which 76 mg contain 1 unit.

Bioassay has some advantages over chemical assay. It is not necessary to know what the active principles are or even to isolate them. It may be exceedingly sensitive and can also be used to assay pure but unstable drugs without loss of activity. There are various ways of doing assays and the *British Pharmacopoeia* gives details of the current official ones.

(i) *Direct assay*. In this method the individual effective dose for each animal is determined by giving the drug till the required effect is obtained. An example is the official assay for digitalis where the drug is administered intravenously to anaesthetized guinea-pigs or pigeons till the heart is arrested. By comparing the volume of the standard and unknown solutions of drugs required to stop the heart in different groups (of the same species), the potency of the unknown preparation can be calculated by a simple proportionate sum. The procedure in the assay is strictly defined, otherwise the comparisons are liable to error.

(ii) *Assays dependent on quantal effects*. Here the occurrence is measured of some easily observed phenomenon such as death or convulsions. The unknown and the standard are given to separate groups of animals and the percentages showing positive effects in each group are compared. An example of this is the assay of insulin by subcutaneous injection into mice when effects such as death or hypoglycaemic coma are described as occurring or not occurring in each animal.

(iii) *Assays dependent on measured or graded effects.* This is the simplest form of assay and the samples of the drug, standard and unknown, are given alternately to the same tissue. If the effects are plotted with the log-dose as abscissa, this gives two parallel straight lines where the horizontal distance apart is proportional to the difference in potency. A common design of the experiment is to give two different doses each of the standard and the unknown (2×2 assay).

Cross-over test. If the effect of the drug can be measured more than once in the same animal, the accuracy of the assay is enhanced by the cross-over test. The animals are divided into two groups and each group is given the standard and the unknown on separate occasions and the results averaged. This eliminates errors due to the animals themselves as each receives the standard and the unknown.

Bioavailability. The way in which the formulation of a drug dosage form may influence the amount and rate of absorption of the active principle has already been discussed (page 6).

THE DEVELOPMENT OF NEW DRUGS

The present era has seen the emergence of many new drugs of varying value. The development of a new drug follows a complex path which usually starts by a pharmaceutical firm synthesizing or isolating substances which are thought to be of potential therapeutic and commercial value either from their structural relationship to known active compounds or from an entirely novel viewpoint. These are extensively studied in animals before deciding to investigate their effects in man. The animal tests attempt to characterize the pharmacological actions of the potential new drug; to compare it with other and established drugs and to determine any toxic effects. A number of different species of animals are used which by previous experience are known to give the most useful information. The drug is used both in acute tests and for prolonged periods to determine the chance of accumulation or long-term effects. The effects of drugs in man are not always the same as in other animals and on occasion may be very different indeed; and no matter how searching the tests on animals are, they still may not show the possibility of some toxic effect which may be seen so rarely that it may take years for the drug to become suspect. The doctor should at all times be alert to the possibility that an unusual symptom in a patient is the unsuspected side effect of a drug.

The drug is also investigated for any potential toxicity to the fetus as the tragic story of thalidomide has brought about an acute sense of awareness of the possible dangers of using any drug in a pregnant woman. It must not be forgotten that it is possible for a woman to become pregnant during the administration of a drug.

These teratogenicity studies are usually carried out in at least 2 species of animals and the drug given during the period of organogenesis. The fetuses are examined for abnormalities or for evidence of their death *in utero*. Investigations must also be made into the possibility of the drug having toxic effects later in pregnancy or during labour and the perinatal period. It must also be determined if the drug has any effects on fertility or on the germ cells.

Various mathematical formulae have been proposed to give some quantitative assessment of the likelihood of a drug giving toxic effects. They are derived mainly from animal experiments and are not necessarily useful in man.

Lethal dose. The Minimum Lethal Dose is the average of the smallest dose that kills and the largest dose that does not kill. The Median Lethal Dose (LD50) is the dose which kills half of a population and is normally expressed as mg of drug/kg animal.

Species differences make these indices useless as guides to the lethal dose in a different species.

Therapeutic index. This is an attempt to measure the therapeutic value of a drug by relating the useful dose to the toxic dose. A therapeutic index proposed by Ehrlich was the ratio maximum tolerated dose:minimum curative dose, but this does not take into account the variability of a normally distributed population and might be better expressed as the $\frac{LD50}{ED50}$. Unlike the therapeutic index of Ehrlich this latter index does not take into account the margin between the safe and effective doses and could be replaced by the $\frac{LD0\cdot1}{ED.999}$ which is the ratio between the dose killing 1 in a 1000 and the dose which would cure all but 1 in 1000.

The Standard Safety Margin. This is the percentage increase above the therapeutic dose which is lethal to a given proportion of subjects. An example of this is phenobarbitone in mice, where the dose producing sleep in 99% has to be increased by 34% before 1% die, and where the dose producing sleep in 99·9% has to be increased by only 8% to be lethal to 1%.

These therapeutic indices are obviously of very limited value in deciding the dose of a drug to be given to man.

Clinical and Therapeutic Trials

If these preliminary animal experiments show *prima facie* evidence that the potential new drug will be of use, the decision has to be made whether to try its effects in man to study its safety, efficacy and toxicity. It must be emphasized that experiments in man are the only way to provide unequivocal evidence of the therapeutic value of the drug in man. The drug is usually given first to normal volunteers to compare its pharmacodynamics and pharmacokinetics with the previous animal studies and to establish possible dosage levels. The drug is then tried in a few selected patients under very carefully controlled conditions by expert physicians who assess its effects in the potential therapeutic situation. This type of study has to be authorized under the Medicines Act (page 3) by a Clinical Trials Certificate.

If these initial clinical studies are satisfactory, the decision has to be made whether to put the drug on general release, i.e. to market it. The manufacturer has to seek permission from the Licensing Authority to do this and only when the relevant Product Licence is issued can he advertise and sell the drug.

A therapeutic trial must be carefully designed beforehand with the aims laid down in every detail as to the type of case to be included and the exact question the trial is designed to answer. It must decide if the new drug is of value especially compared with drugs already in use and the type of patient and administration best suited for the drug.

In principle, the health of the treated patient is compared with untreated patients though sometimes the patient may act as his own control as in generalized skin disease or in steady state chronic disease.

It is important that the groups compared should be equivalent in every way save for the control group not having the treatment. This includes age, sex, social class and severity of disease. They should also be compared concurrently, which may raise considerable ethical problems if a new and apparently life-saving drug is being investigated. The historical control, where the past records of the pre-new drug days are used as controls, is a bad method.

It is also preferable to use the double blind technique where, in order to prevent bias from influencing the result, the drug or dummy is given to the patient (first blind man) and his progress is assessed by someone (second blind man) who does not know what the patient has had.

It is necessary to apply statistical tests of significance to a therapeutic trial to assess the probability that the observations are due to chance and for details of the methods used, a textbook of statistics should be consulted.

The use of therapeutic trials is not to deny the value of opinion about individual cases but this is usually too subjective to allow of generalizations.

Many trials in widely different places and some years of experience of the drug are usually necessary before permitting generalized use and acceptance.

Placebos (Lat. *placere*, please). In the subjective assessment of the condition of a patient on treatment, suggestibility plays a large part and must always be borne in mind when assessing the effects of a drug. This placebo effect may occur even if the drug is potent and cures the condition, though preparations may be given as frank placebos either for the benefit of the patient or perhaps for the doctor himself. The placebo is not a special kind of preparation and there is an art in choosing the particular formulation to suit the patient. It is estimated that 30% or so of the population are placebo reactors to a varying degree. There appears to be a definite psychological type involved but it is not easy to distinguish this without special testing. Some subjects may be negative placebo reactors and notice unfavourable reactions.

Adverse Drug Effects in Man

Although when talking about receptors the selective action of drugs was discussed, this selectivity is relative and drugs usually have more than one action. It seems reasonable to maintain that any given action of a drug is wanted or not wanted. The main action is that desired therapeutically or pharmacologically.

The unwanted effects range from the trivial to the fatal and are sometimes difficult to define, and the terms unwanted effect, side effect, toxic effect, adverse effect may mean the same or be very different according to the person using them. These unwanted actions arise from a variety of causes. They may be due to other known and expected actions of the drug when they are often called side effects. However, these same side effects may on another occasion be the wanted effects, as for example the sedation caused by the competitive antihistamines (see page 39). Sometimes the wanted pharmacological actions of the drug cause indirectly an unwanted effect (secondary effect), and a typical example of this is the infection of the gut (superinfection) caused by the overgrowth of resistant organisms when a patient is given an oral broad-spectrum antibiotic.

Some of the unwanted effects of a drug may be the exaggerated normal ones, perhaps with secondary consequences. This is especially likely to occur with an overdose of the drug taken either acutely or when it has accumulated to toxic levels.

Idiosyncrasy (Gk. *idios*, own; *sun*, with; *krasis*, combination). This is an apparently abnormal response to the drug and is usually due to some abnormal mechanism by which the drug is handled. A typical example is the occasional person who lacks the pseudo-cholinesterase to metabolize suxamethonium. This may cause a paralysis of respiration (suxamethonium apnoea). To some, idiosyncrasy means an allergic response but this is better called hypersensitivity.

Hypersensitivity (Gk. *huper*, over; Lat. *sentire*, to feel). This is an altered reactivity to a drug which acts as an antigen and causes antigen–antibody reactions. Some have used it to mean one end of the normal variation in the response of a population to a dose of a drug though this is usually referred to as intolerance.

Intolerance. This is said to occur when the normal and characteristic effect is seen in unusually small doses. It is a reflection of the normal variation seen in any population.

Dependence and Addiction. These are discussed on page 236.

Teratogenicity. This is discussed on page 34.

Drug–drug interactions ('pharmacokinetic interactions')

A drug can modify significantly the action or effect of another when administered concurrently and because patients are commonly treated with several drugs simultaneously over long periods it is important to consider the possible consequences of such polypharmacy. Quite often this may be simple antagonism or synergism at the site of action (page 21) but the interactions can be more complex and although examples will be discussed with the individual drugs it is as well to list the possible types and to remember the likelihood of such an occurrence when using multiple drug therapy or to explain an unexpected side effect. These interactions may conveniently be listed under the major heading of Chapter 2 which discusses the concentration of a drug at its site of action, i.e. absorption, distribution, biotransformation and excretion. For reasons of space, only one or two examples of each type are given and the list must under no circumstances be thought complete as the number of possible combinations is vast. In many cases, of course, the drug–drug interaction is desirable and sought for therapeutically, e.g. nalorphine in morphine overdose (page 134). Interactions between drugs may also occur in their preparation and mixtures should not be made extemporaneously unless compatibility is certain. Thiopentone and suxamethonium, for example, interact chemically and must not be put together in the same syringe.

(i) *Absorption*. Most drugs have to be absorbed to give an effective concentration at the site of action (page 4) and many factors influence this. Changes in gut pH (e.g. antacids, page 245) will affect the absorption of some drugs such as salicylates (page 5). Absorption may also be influenced by the excipient used to give bulk to tablets (page 6). Changes in gastric motility (e.g. by atropine-like drugs, pages 50, 97) may have important influences on absorption especially if gastric emptying is delayed. Absorption of tetracyclines is greatly lessened by the concomitant administration of iron (e.g. for anaemia) or of calcium, magnesium and aluminium (e.g. as antacids).

(ii) *Distribution*. Many drugs are protein bound in the plasma (page 11) and as some appear to have common binding sites whose number is limited, one drug may displace another. Although the displacement may seem small in total amount, it must be remembered that it is the unbound drug which is the active moiety and even slight displacements can cause the proportion of unbound drug to rise sharply. If, for example, a drug is normally 95% bound (i.e. 5% of the total drug is unbound and active) and has only 5% displaced, the amount of unbound drug doubles and consequently the activity. A classical example is the displacement of the anticoagulant warfarin from its binding site by aspirin, phenylbutazone, indomethacin or clofibrate with a consequent gross decrease in the coagulability of the blood.

(iii) *Metabolism.* The intensity and duration of action of many drugs is related to the rate of biotransformation to inactive compounds. This conversion is normally made by liver enzymes. Many drugs stimulate the formation of these enzymes ('enzyme induction', page 13) and consequently the rate of their own metabolism and that of other drugs similarly affected. This may make the dosage schedule of many drugs unsuitable if the inducing agent is stopped. A typical example is the induction of liver enzymes caused by barbiturates which also increases the rate of biotransformation of coumarin-type anticoagulants. If the barbiturate is withdrawn and the anticoagulant schedule not modified, when the effect of induction wears off (2–3 weeks) the rate of metabolism of the coumarin drugs falls and the coagulability of the blood may drop to dangerous and even fatal levels.

Many drugs also inhibit drug metabolism though this is not so well documented as stimulation. A good example is the block of ethanol metabolism by disulfiram (page 209).

(iv) *Excretion.* Non-protein bound drugs and their metabolites are filtered at the glomerulus but may be reabsorbed in the tubules dependent on pH and lipid solubility. Changes in urinary pH will therefore alter the excretion rate of many drugs (page 177) and consequently their degree and duration of action. Many acidic drugs (e.g. salicylic acid, sulphonamides, phenylbutazone, indomethacin, thiazide diuretics, chlorpropamide) are actively secreted by the renal tubules and competition may arise for this system (e.g. penicillin and probenecid, page 263).

REFERENCES

Burn, J. H., Finney, D. J. & Goodwin, L. G. (1950) *Biological Standardization*, 2nd edn. Oxford University Press.

Finney, D. J. (1964) *Statistical Methods in Biological Assay*, 2nd edn. London: Griffin.

Harris, E. L. & Fitzgerald, J. D. (eds.) (1970) *The Principles and Practice of Clinical Trials*. Edinburgh: Livingstone.

Martin, E. W. (ed.) (1971) *Hazards of Medication*. Oxford: Blackwell.

Meyler, L. & Herxheimer, A. (eds.) (1972) *Side Effects of Drugs*. Vol. VII. Amsterdam: Excerpta Medica Foundation.

Turner, R. A. (1965) *Screening Methods in Pharmacology*. London: Academic Press.

The British Pharmacopoeia 1973.

5   The Autonomic Nervous System I

INTRODUCTION

The autonomic nervous system consists of the splanchnic or visceral components of the nervous system with fibres distributed to the various viscera, glands, blood vessels and smooth muscle. It has both parasympathetic and sympathetic divisions, each with motor and sensory fibres, and is under the control of the central nervous system at medullary (the vital centres), thalamic and cortical levels. Much of the autonomic nervous system, however, can function in isolation. The effects of stimulating the autonomic nerves in man are briefly summarized in Table I.

Autonomic Transmission

It was shown early this century that transmission of the nerve impulse across the synaptic gap to the effector cell was due to the release of chemical substances, and Dale in 1933 proposed that the nomenclature of fibres in the nervous system be divided as regards the chemical transmission of their activity without regard to their anatomical connections.

1. Cholinergic fibres

These nerves release acetylcholine at their terminals. They include all autonomic preganglionic fibres, all parasympathetic post-ganglionic fibres, sympathetic nerve endings to the adrenal medulla (which embryologically is a ganglion) and sympathetic

41

TABLE I. The effect of stimulating the autonomic nerves in man

Tissue	Adrenergic Nerves	Cholinergic Nerves
1. *Heart*		
Rate:	Increased	Decreased
Stroke volume:	Increased	Decreased
2. *Blood vessels*		
(a) *arterioles*		
Coronary:	Dilated	
Skin:	Constricted	
Skeletal muscle:	Dilated/Constricted	
Cerebral:	Constricted	
Pulmonary	Constricted	
Visceral:	Constricted	
(b) *Veins*	Constricted	
3. *Stomach and intestine*		
Mobility and tone:	Decreased	Increased
Sphincters:	Constricted	Relaxed
Secretions:	Inhibited	Increased
4. *Respiratory tract*		
Bronchial muscle:	Relaxed	Constricted
5. *Urinary tract*		
Bladder tone:	Decreased	Increased
Bladder sphincter:	Constricted	Relaxed
Ureter tone:	Decreased	Increased
6. *Uterus*	Variable	Variable
7. *Eye*		
Iris:	Dilated	Constricted
Ciliary muscle:	Relaxed for far vision	Accommodated for near vision
8. *Skin*		
Pilomotor muscle:	Contracted	
9. *Liver*	Glycogenolysis	
10. *Glands*		
Sweat:		Secretion
Bronchial:		Secretion
Lacrimal:		Secretion
Salivary:	Sparse mucous secretion	Profuse watery secretion

cholinergic nerve endings to some sweat glands and blood vessels. The somatic nerves to skeletal muscle are also cholinergic.

Muscarine-like and nicotine-like actions. The actions of acetylcholine may be further divided into the muscarine-like (muscarinic) and the nicotine-like (nicotinic). The muscarine-like actions,

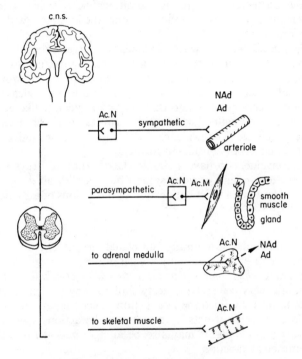

FIG. 5. Chemical transmitters in the nervous system.
    Ac.N nicotine-like action of acetylcholine
    Ac.M muscarine-like action of acetylcholine
    N.Ad noradrenaline
    Ad   adrenaline

so called because they resemble those of the alkaloid muscarine, are equivalent to the actions of acetylcholine at parasympathetic post-ganglionic endings. They are blocked by atropine and enhanced by anticholinesterases. The nicotine-like actions resemble the stimulant actions of nicotine and are equivalent to the actions of acetylcholine at the autonomic ganglia and the neuromuscular junction. They are not blocked by atropine but are blocked by the various ganglion and neuromuscular junction-blocking drugs.

2. Adrenergic fibres

These are nerves which release noradrenaline at their terminals. They include all post-ganglionic sympathetic fibres with the exceptions mentioned above.

This simple picture, where cholinergic nerves release acetylcholine and adrenergic nerves release noradrenaline, is illustrated in Fig. 5. It has been complicated in recent years by the work of Burn and others who say that acetylcholine is also released at adrenergic nerve endings and that this, by a nicotine-like action, releases noradrenaline which then causes the characteristic adrenergic effects. The evidence for this theory is not universally accepted and is not considered further.

It is convenient to have a simple classification of drugs which affect the autonomic nervous system but, as with all drugs, this is a guide and not a strict delineation of the actions of a particular drug.

(i) *Drugs with acetylcholine-like effects.* These include choline esters; alkaloids structurally unrelated to acetylcholine but having similar effects; and anticholinesterases.

(ii) *Drugs which antagonize the action of acetylcholine.* In the autonomic nervous system, acetylcholine may be antagonized where it acts by nicotine-like actions such as at autonomic ganglia and where it acts by muscarine-like actions such as on the heart and glands. It may also be antagonized at the skeletal neuromuscular junction.

(iii) *Drugs with noradrenaline-like effects.* These may be considered either under chemical structure or by their mode of action on the adrenergic mechanisms. Drugs which exert some or all of the effects of stimulating the sympathetic system are sometimes described as sympathomimetic.

(iv) *Drugs which antagonize the adrenergic mechanisms.* This may be antagonized either by blocking the adrenergic receptor (adrenergic receptor blocking drug) or by blocking the release of the adrenergic transmitter from the nerve ending (adrenergic neurone-blocking drug).

Transmission in the central nervous system

This is a controversial subject and many compounds have been implicated by various workers in different parts of the central nervous system. They include acetylcholine, noradrenaline, adrenaline, dopamine, 5-hydroxytryptamine, glutamine, gamma amino butyric acid and ergothionine. Many drugs may act on some of these putative central transmitters and are discussed under the appropriate headings.

REFERENCES

Burn, J. H. (1971) *The Autonomic Nervous System*, 4th edn. Oxford: Blackwell Scientific Publications.

Dale, Sir Henry H. (1965) *Adventures in Physiology*. London: The Wellcome Trust.

6

The Autonomic Nervous System II

ACETYLCHOLINE-LIKE DRUGS

These act at some or all of the following sites: nicotinic sites (such as the ganglia and the neuromuscular junction); at muscarinic sites (parasympathetic and some sympathetic post-ganglionic endings); and at some sites in the central nervous system.

1. Acetylcholine

The formation of acetylcholine is discussed on page 78 with the neuromuscular junction, but a similar process probably occurs at other sites. Structurally acetylcholine is an onium compound, i.e. a substance where an alkyl or more elaborate radical has replaced the hydrogens of the ammonium ion (though the term may be extended to other ionic centres such as phosphonium and stibonium). Choline, the parent compound, was discovered by Strecker in 1849 in pig bile and has weak and unimportant cholinergic actions.

Acetylcholine is rapidly hydrolysed by cholinesterases (page 47) and has a very transient action. It is not effective orally, intramuscularly or subcutaneously. The divisions of the actions of acetylcholine into muscarine-like and nicotine-like have already been discussed, but they are too brief for acetylcholine to be of use in therapy. Other onium compounds may act similarly to acetylcholine, but if there is no ester link they will not be so rapidly hydrolysed by cholinesterases. Variations in structure may also produce different affinities for different tissues.

2. Methacholine (Acetyl Methyl Choline)

This choline ester has predominantly muscarine-like actions, particularly those on the cardiovascular system. It is destroyed only slowly by cholinesterases (but not by pseudocholinesterase). It may be given parenterally and orally, though is somewhat unreliable by this latter route.

3. Carbachol (Carbamoyl Choline)

This is a choline ester not destroyed by cholinesterases and stable enough to be given orally or by injection. It has both muscarine-like and nicotine-like actions and stimulates the gut and bladder and also causes salivation, nausea and sweating. It is used to stimulate the intestine in ileus; in paroxysmal tachycardia; or in atonic non-obstructive retention of urine.

4. Pilocarpine

This compound has an action similar to that of acetylcholine, but is an alkaloid and so is not destroyed by cholinesterases. It acts especially on those sweat glands which are cholinergic in innervation and on the salivary, bronchial and gastric glands. It stimulates and then depresses the central nervous system and has only slight action at the neuromuscular junction and ganglia. It is used therapeutically to reduce the intraocular pressure in glaucoma.

5. Muscarine

This compound occurs in the mushroom fly agaric (*Amanita muscaria*) and gives its name to the muscarine-like actions it produces.

6. Anticholinesterases

These drugs inhibit or inactivate cholinesterases and so prevent the destruction of acetylcholine which will potentiate its effects.

Acetylcholine is removed from its site of action by diffusion and hydrolysis. This latter action is catalysed by cholinesterases of which there are two kinds. True cholinesterase is specific for acetylcholine (acetylcholinesterase) and is found especially at synapses and in red cells. True cholinesterase will also hydrolyse other choline esters and some non-choline esters such as acetate. Pseudocholinesterase (butyrylcholinesterase) is found especially in the plasma and the intestinal mucosa and plays little part in the hydrolysis of endogenous acetylcholine and its normal substrate is unknown. It will also destroy such esters as procaine and suxamethonium.

A cholinesterase has an active site with an anionic (nitrogen attracting) and an esteratic (ester binding) subsites. Acetylcholine, for example, forms a reversible enzyme-substrate complex followed by acetylation of the esteratic subsite and release of choline. The acetylated acetylcholinesterase is very unstable and quickly splits to form the free enzyme and acetic acid.

The action of anticholinesterases is to compete with substrates for the active sites of cholinesterase and so to interfere with the hydrolysis of these substances. This will promote the accumulation of acetylcholine and so augment both muscarine-like and nicotine-like activity.

The competition by anticholinesterases may be reversible or non-reversible. The reversible anticholinesterases form an analogous complex to acetylcholine, but hydrolysis is very much slower thus effectively blocking the hydrolysis of acetylcholine. In non-reversible inhibition caused by anticholinesterases such as the organophosphates, an enzyme complex is formed which is stable and no regeneration of the enzyme occurs, so cholinesterase activity returns only when new enzyme is synthesized.

(a) Physostigmine (eserine)

This drug is an alkaloid obtained from the calabar bean and is a lipid soluble tertiary amine. It is a reversible inhibitor of cholinesterases with a predominance of muscarine-like effects. It is excitant on the central nervous system as it can penetrate the blood–brain barrier. It is well absorbed orally and may be used topically on the conjunctiva (page 75).

(b) Neostigmine

This is a synthetic quaternary ammonium compound readily absorbed parenterally but poorly by mouth and passes the blood-brain barrier very slowly. It is destroyed in the liver and excreted via the urine. It is a reversible inhibitor of cholinesterases with a predominance of nicotine-like effects. It has also a direct stimulant action on the pre-synaptic segment of the neuromuscular junction facilitating repetitive discharge. It is used for its muscarine-like actions in the treatment of paralytic ileus and glaucoma. It is used for its nicotine-like action in myasthenia gravis (page 84) and to antagonize curare-like drugs (page 79).

(c) Organophosphorus compounds

Organic esters of phosphoric acid are powerful inhibitors of cholinesterases and also inhibit other enzymes. They form a phosphorylated enzyme complex which is extremely stable. Virtually no hydrolysis occurs and cholinesterase activity returns only when new enzyme is formed.

(i) *Dyflos (di-isopropylfluorophosphonate, DFP)*. This compound forms an enzyme complex which is stable for a week or more. It causes a powerful and prolonged constriction of the pupil if applied locally and is used as long-acting miotic in glaucoma.

(ii) *Various*. Other organophosphates include the insecticides parathion, mipafox and TEPP (ethylpyrophosphate); the nerve gas sarin; and ecothiopate which is used to treat glaucoma.

Anticholinesterase poisoning

Poisoning may easily occur with anticholinesterases either accidentally or intentionally due to their use as insecticides or war gases. The symptoms are those of excessive muscarine-like and nicotine-like actions. Atropine will antagonize the muscarine-like symptoms and the competitive neuromuscular-blocking drugs and ganglion-blocking drugs have some antidotal effect to the nicotine-like actions.

Recently, derivatives of hydroxamic acid have been made such as pralidoxime mesylate (P2S) which have a high affinity for phosphoryl groups and will compete with cholinesterases for them. By this means it may be possible to reactivate cholinesterases poisoned by organophosphates. Unfortunately, the phosphorylated cholinesterase rapidly loses its ability to be reactivated by the oximes. This ageing is caused by loss of an alkyl group from the phosphorylated enzyme to form an even more stable compound. The rate of ageing varies from a few minutes to several days, dependent on the particular compound.

ANTAGONISTS OF ACETYLCHOLINE

The actions of acetylcholine may be antagonized at three main sites: the muscarine-like actions at post-ganglionic cholinergic nerve endings; the nicotine-like actions at autonomic ganglia; and at the neuromuscular junction.

Antagonists of the Muscarine-like Actions of Acetylcholine

These block the post-synaptic membrane of cells innervated by post-ganglionic cholinergic fibres. The mechanism is by competition for the active site (competitive antagonism). They do not prevent the liberation of acetylcholine but occupy the receptors and so prevent triggering of the muscarine-like actions. There are minor differences between members of this group of drugs due, perhaps, to different degrees of affinity.

1. Atropine (racemic or dl-hyoscyamine)

This drug is found in plants belonging to the family *Solanaceae* such as Deadly Nightshade (*Atropa belladonna*), probably as the separate isomers, though racemization occurs easily. The laevo-isomer, hyoscyamine, is the active isomer, being some twenty times more potent than the dextro form. Atropine is readily absorbed orally and parenterally and has the following actions:

(i) It is a competitive antagonist of the muscarine-like actions of acetylcholine, though they are not all equally affected by atropine. Salivation is very sensitive and atropine readily causes a dry mouth. Bronchial and sweat secretions are similarly reduced even with very small doses of atropine. The vagus and the oculo-motor nuclei are less sensitive and the parasympathetic supply to the gut and bladder even less so. The nervous phase of gastric secretion is the least sensitive of all.

(ii) Atropine produces a stimulant and then depressant effect on the central nervous system, which is usually seen only when an overdose is taken.

Therapeutic uses of atropine. Atropine and the atropine-like drugs are much used in therapeutics. On the eye, atropine causes mydriasis and blocks accommodation (page 76). Preoperatively, atropine may form part of the premedication given to patients to block the secretion of mucus in the respiratory tract and to abolish vagal reflexes (page 220). Atropine and the atropine-like drugs may be used as spasmolytics, that is drugs which lessen the frequency and force of smooth muscle contraction (page 97) and also in the treatment of peptic ulcer (page 247).

2. Homatropine

This drug is synthetic and has a similar action to that of atropine though with only 10% of the potency. It is often preferred for use in the eye as the actions are quicker in onset but shorter in duration, lasting about 12–24 hours compared to those of atropine which may last a week or more. It has little other use.

3. Hyoscine

Hyoscine is found chiefly in the leaves of the plant *Hyoscyamus niger*. It has a similar though briefer effect to atropine on muscarine-like actions, which when compared with atropine, is quantitatively stronger on the iris, ciliary muscle and exocrine glands, though less so on the vagus, intestine and bronchioles. Hyoscine is, however, a central nervous depressant and not a stimulant like atropine though it may cause excitation in the elderly.

It is used to prevent motion sickness by its sedative action and is very effective. It is also used to suppress unwanted secretions during anaesthesia and to reduce the skeletal muscle rigidity of paralysis agitans. Although sedative, hyoscine has no analgesic action and stimulates rather than depresses respiration.

The side effects are those of unwanted anti-muscarine-like actions such as dry mouth, loss of accommodation and difficulty in micturition.

Parkinsonism

This syndrome, first described by Parkinson in 1817, is characterized by rigidity, tremor and hypokinesia. The aetiology is varied and the types include the post-encephalitic, arteriosclerotic or induced by drugs such as reserpine, phenothiazines and the butyrophenones.

Histologically the most characteristic finding is a fall in the dopamine content of the corpus striatum and the substantia nigra (the 'nigro-striatal' pathway). Cholinergic fibres to the striatum appear unimpaired and there seems to be a relative imbalance of the cholinergic and dopaminergic pathways. Parkinsonism is worsened by substances which increase acetylcholine levels and improved by substances which either antagonize acetylcholine or increase dopamine levels.

(i) *Anticholinergic drugs.* The use of atropine and hyoscine has been replaced by synthetic drugs such as benzhexol, orphenadrine, benztropine. These drugs are effective in relieving rigidity and tremor but not hypokinesia. They are also effective in relieving drug-induced Parkinsonism which is more likely to be due to a block of dopaminergic receptors than an absolute deficiency of dopamine, hence increasing dopamine per se will be of little value. The side effects of the anticholinergic drugs are those of parasympathetic block such as impaired accommodation, dry mouth and some central nervous effects such as confusion and hallucinations.

(ii) *Amantadine.* This antiviral drug (see page 274) improves all three major features of Parkinsonism, the tremor, the rigidity and the hypokinesia. Its mode of action is not known but is probably by dopamine release.

(iii) *Levodopa* (L-dopa). Dopamine itself does not cross the blood–brain barrier to a useful degree though its precursor levodopa (see page 58) will do so and result in an increase in the level of brain dopamine. Conversion of levodopa to dopamine also occurs peripherally.

Levodopa is the most potent drug available against Parkinsonism and causes a dramatic clinical improvement in a high proportion of patients. Nausea, vomiting and postural hypotension may occur in the early stages of treatment. During long-term administration, rapid but transient deteriorations may occur and there may also be endocrine disturbances due to dopamine mediated pituitary release.

GANGLION-BLOCKING DRUGS

Transmission at the autonomic ganglion resembles that at the neuromuscular junction, and when a nerve impulse reaches the end of the preganglionic fibre, acetylcholine is released to cause a depolarization of the post-ganglionic fibre and the propagation of the impulse. All preganglionic fibres, both sympathetic and parasympathetic, are therefore cholinergic and this action of acetylcholine is a nicotine-like one. Like the neuromuscular junction, small spontaneous potentials can be recorded from the post-synaptic membrane and it seems probable that these can summate to cause a full ganglionic spike potential.

Certain drugs prevent the transmission of the nerve impulse across the ganglion. Some may interfere with the synthesis or release of acetylcholine such as hemicholinium, botulinus toxin, a low calcium or a high magnesium concentration. Some drugs such as hexamethonium may compete with acetylcholine for the receptor sites on the post-synaptic membrane, occupying them but not causing depolarization (non-depolarizing or competitive block). Some drugs such as nicotine cause the post-synaptic membrane to become insensitive to released acetylcholine, perhaps after an initial stimulation, a so-called depolarization or densensitization block.

Ganglionic-blocking drugs such as hexamethonium and pentolinium are quaternary ammonium compounds and are wholly ionized when in solution. They are therefore poorly absorbed from the gastrointestinal tract and have to be given parenterally. Non-quaternary compounds such as mecamylamine and pempidine are well absorbed by mouth, which is a great advantage therapeutically.

The Effects of the Ganglion-blocking Drugs

(i) *Circulation.* The major effect on the circulation is due to interference with the sympathetic vasoconstrictor pathways. The effect on the arterial blood pressure depends on the normal pressure, posture, and the presence of other drugs. As the blood pressure is dependent on the cardiac output and the total peripheral resistance; hypotension will result if the latter is decreased by interrupting vasomotor tone to the arterioles and venous bed.

This hypotension will be greater in the upright position (postural or orthostatic hypotension) due to the interference with compensatory reflex paths. This interference also makes the circulation very sensitive to pressor agents such as noradrenaline.

(ii) *Alimentary tract.* Salivary and gastric secretions will be depressed and the response to insulin abolished as it is mediated through the vagus though the direct response to histamine persists. Motor activity is also depressed and ileus or constipation may result.

(iii) *The eye.* Moderate dilatation of the pupil occurs, as normally the parasympathetic tone is greater than the sympathetic, and when both are completely paralysed, constriction is affected proportionately more. Accommodation is also paralysed and vision may be blurred.

(iv) *Various effects.* Sweating is decreased and the skin is warm due to peripheral vasodilatation which could cause the body temperature to fall. Other effects include paralysis of the bladder, impotence and dryness of the mouth.

The Uses of the Ganglion-blocking Drugs

Their major use is to decrease blood pressure as this may be of benefit in the treatment of hypertension (page 149). They do not cure the hypertension but the fall in blood pressure may relieve the clinical symptoms and prolong life. The ganglion-blocking drugs act on both the parasympathetic and sympathetic ganglia and it is important to remember that there are no ganglion-blocking drugs which block the sympathetic ganglia and leave the parasympathetic ganglia unimpaired. The unwanted side effects of constipation, ileus, dry mouth, paralysis of accommodation and of interference with the functioning of the bladder and the sex act are grave drawbacks to their use in the treatment of hypertension and they have largely been replaced by other drugs, though there is still a place for them in anaesthetic practice and in the emergency reduction of blood pressure.

Individual Ganglion-blocking Drugs

1. *Nicotine.* This is an alkaloid obtained from the tobacco plant. It is readily absorbed from all mucous membranes, subcutaneously and even from the intact skin. Its actions give the

name to the nicotine-like effects of acetylcholine. It excites then depresses the central nervous system and causes a release of vasopressin (antidiuretic hormone). It paralyses all autonomic ganglia after an initial stimulation to cause a depolarization type of block. Sympathetic effects include a rise in blood pressure and heart rate due to stimulation of the adrenal medulla. In tobacco smoking the parasympathetic effects of slow pulse, nausea, vomiting and increase in tone and motor activity of the bowel may be the most obvious. Nicotine also stimulates neuromuscular transmission and fasciculation of skeletal muscle may result.

2. *The bis-quaternary ammonium series.* The compound illustrated in the diagram is the basic structure of the bis-quaternary

$$(CH_3)_3.N\text{------}(CH_2)_n\text{------}N.(CH_3)_3$$

The basic structure of the bis-quaternary ammonium series

ammonium series (bisonium compounds) and forms an interesting example of structure-activity relationships. If in the methylene chain, n = 5 (pentamethonium) or 6 (hexamethonium) then ganglion-blocking activity predominates. If n = 9 or 10 (decamethonium) then neuromuscular-blocking activity occurs. *Hexamethonium*: as this drug is a quaternary ammonium compound it is ionized in solution and so is poorly absorbed from the gut and must be given parenterally. It produces a brief and reversible ganglion block, though in high doses it also has an atropine and curare-like action.

It is distributed through the extracellular fluid and is excreted via the kidney unchanged. It is little used these days save in anaesthetic practise and as an emergency treatment of hypertensive crises.

3. *Mecamylamine.* This drug is a secondary amine which is rapidly and completely absorbed by mouth. The action is slow in onset and sustained as the drug penetrates intracellularly and becomes bound to protein. It both crosses the placenta and enters the cerebrospinal fluid. Excretion is also slow and mainly via the urine. It is slowed more if the urine is alkaline, in which mecamylamine is predominantly non-ionized, and is increased if the urine is acid. This could be of importance if other drugs were given such as chlorothiazide which change the reaction of the urine.

The side effects are those of ganglion blockade especially ileus and constipation. Central nervous effects can occur such as tremor, confusion and delirium.

4. *Pempidine.* This drug is a tertiary amine and like mecamylamine is also well absorbed by mouth. It is also quickly excreted as it is not so protein bound as mecamylamine. It has typical ganglion-blocking effects and also a weak neuromuscular-blocking action.

REFERENCES

Goodman, L. S. & Gilman, A. (1975) *The Pharmacological Basis of Therapeutics,* 5th edn. Baillière Tindall : London, New York: Macmillan.

Hobbiger, F. (1968) Anticholinesterases. In *Recent Advances in Pharmacology,* 4th edn. Robson, J. M. & Stacey, R. S. (eds.). pp. 281–310. London: Churchill.

7

The Autonomic Nervous System III

THE ADRENERGIC NEURONE

The post-ganglionic fibres of the sympathetic nervous system are mainly adrenergic, i.e. the transmitter liberated at the nerve ending is noradrenaline with perhaps some adrenaline. A very few post-ganglionic sympathetic fibres, which go to some sweat glands and blood vessels, are cholinergic and liberate acetylcholine at their endings.

The current concept of the adrenergic nerve fibre is that the nerve impulse causes depolarization and increased permeability to calcium which enters the cell and causes the release of noradrenaline and a little adrenaline from the nerve terminal. There is some evidence, as has been mentioned previously, that all post-ganglionic fibres first release acetylcholine and then this (by a nicotine-like action) releases noradrenaline from the adrenergic fibre.

Noradrenaline, adrenaline and dopamine are members of the catecholamine group of compounds (catechol is dihydroxybenzene). These are distributed throughout the tissues in cells called chromaffin cells due to the brown colour produced when they are treated with dichromate, though the presence of catecholamines may be more elegantly shown by fluorescence techniques. The actual percentage of the various catecholamines in the chromaffin cells depends on the site and the species. In the gut, it is mainly dopamine which occurs in non-nerve cells. There is very little dopamine in the adrenal medulla but there is a lot of adrenaline. In other organs and probably in association with nerve fibres,

57

dopamine accounts for about half of the catecholamines content, the rest being noradrenaline with traces of adrenaline.

Dopamine is present in the central grey matter of the brain, especially the caudate nucleus and probably has a transmitter function there. In Parkinsonian patients the dopamine content of the caudate nucleus falls.

The catecholamines are formed mainly along the pathway shown in table II. The rate-limiting reaction is the formation of dopa from tyrosine by tyrosine hydroxylase which is the first step of catecholamine synthesis in chromaffin and adrenergic

TABLE II. Pathway of formation of the catecholamines.

Substrate	Enzyme Reaction	Inhibitors
L-PHENYLALANINE		
↓		
L-TYROSINE	Hydroxylation by tyrosine hydroxylase	a methyl tyrosine 3.iodotyrosine
	Rate-limiting step	
L-DOPA	Decarboxylation by dopa decarboxylase	methyldopa
DOPAMINE	Hydroxylation by dopamine β hydroxylase	disulfiram guanoclor
NORADRENALINE	Methylation by phenylethanolamine-N.methyl transferase	
↓		
ADRENALINE		

tissue. Tyrosine hydroxylase is inhibited by methyltyrosine which reduces the excretion of catecholamine metabolites to about 30% but has no useful antihypertensive action save in phaeochromocytoma. Methyldopa, which inhibits the decarboxylation of dopa by dopa decarboxylase, is discussed on page 69. Dopamine is the first pharmacologically active compound though has only weak pressor actions.

Most of the catecholamines are present in membrane-limited

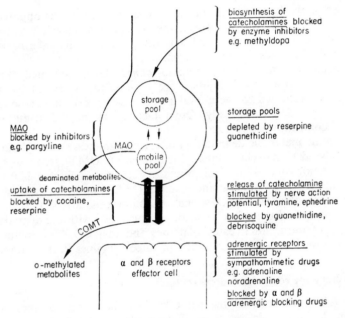

FIG. 6. The adrenergic nerve ending.

subcellular particles called chromaffin granules, though a percentage (20%–40%) appears to be free in the cytoplasm. The granules have a high ATP content, which is in combination with the catecholamines in a 1:4 ratio. There is also a soluble protein (chromogranin), lipid, Ca^{++}, and Mg^{++}. The mechanism of secretion of the catecholamines is in dispute but the evidence seems to favour liberation by exocytosis. The granule membrane fuses with the plasmalemma of the cell and discharges its contents, though not the granular membrane itself, through an aperture in the fused membrane without the contents coming into contact with the cell cytoplasm. The mechanism is calcium dependent and this ion may play an essential role in the fusion of the two membranes.

There is evidence for a similar mechanism of calcium dependent secretion by exocytosis in many different kinds of cells including endocrine and exocrine glands, the mast cell and polymorphonuclear leucocyte.

Some workers feel that in the adrenergic neurone, as opposed to chromaffin tissue elsewhere, the free pool of catecholamines plays an important part and it is from this pool that the nerve impulse liberates the neurotransmitter.

Metabolic fate of the catecholamines. Once liberated, the actions of the catecholamines are terminated in several ways. Most is returned to the granular pool (re-uptake), though some is degraded enzymatically. Other factors include redistribution and compensatory reflexes.

In the metabolic degradation of catecholamines, o-methylation catalysed by catechol-o-methyl transferase (COMT) seems to be the major route with other processes occurring such as oxidative deamination by monoamine oxidases (MAO) or by conjugation. It is probable that MAO, which occurs intracellularly in the outer membrane of the mitochondrion, is concerned with the degradation of intracellular catecholamines and that COMT is mainly concerned with the degradation of catecholamines in the blood.

Adrenergic receptors (adrenoceptors)

After release from the nerve ending, the catecholamines act on the adrenergic receptors of the effector cell. These receptors were defined by Ahlquist in 1948 as '... those hypothetical structures or systems located in, on, or near the muscles or gland cells affected by adrenaline (or noradrenaline)'.

Noradrenaline and adrenaline have a variety of actions which are divided into α and β actions produced by stimulation of the appropriate receptor. These actions are listed in Table III. It will be seen that the α actions are mainly excitatory and α receptors are typically stimulated by noradrenaline which does, however, have some β actions.

The β actions are mainly inhibitory and typically produced by isoprenaline which has very little α actions. Adrenaline has mainly β actions but also some α actions.

TABLE III. Effects of stimulation of the adrenergic receptor

α-Receptors	β-Receptors
Vasoconstriction ((cutaneous, renal, etc.)	β_1-receptors
	Increased heart rate,
Splenic capsule contraction	contractility and excitability
Pilomotor contraction	β_2-receptors
Nictitating membrane contraction	Vasodilatation (skeletal muscle,
Dilator pupillae contraction	coronary bed, etc.)
Bladder sphincter contraction	Bronchial relaxation
Salivary gland secretion	
	uncertain
	Glycogenolysis
	Lipolysis

β actions on the heart, however, are those of stimulation, not inhibition and cause an increase of rate and amplitude of contraction. Some workers have, therefore, divided the β receptors into the β_1 receptors (heart muscle, intestinal smooth muscle) and the β_2 receptors (tracheobronchial muscle, uterus, skeletal muscle arteries). Lipolysis may be a β_1 function and glycogenolysis a β_2 function. Some drugs such as salbutamol (page 66) do show a high degree of selectivity for the different β receptors and, indeed, further subdivision is likely eventually.

The sites of the adrenergic receptors are made obvious by the adrenergic receptor blocking drugs (page 71) which combine with the specific receptor, either α or β, thus not permitting the usual response to be triggered.

The actual mechanism whereby the transmitter produces effects at the effector site is disputed. There are changes in the permeability of the cell membrane of smooth muscle which if it becomes depolarized would lead to the propagation of action potentials and contraction. On the other hand, if the membrane becomes hyperpolarized then the cell becomes more stable and relaxes. The major part of the positive inotropic effect on the heart, for example, is not accounted for by ionic changes and it seems likely that the primary action of β-stimulants is to activate an adenylcyclase which promotes the formation of 3'5'-adenosine monophosphate (cyclic AMP) from ATP. This cyclic AMP then activates a phosphorylase system which accelerates glycogenolysis and thus facilitates energy mobilization.

THE SYMPATHOMIMETIC AMINES

Noradrenaline is derived from phenylethylamine, and a large series of related substances may be formed by substitution in the catechol nucleus (dihydroxybenzene) or the side chain (see diagram). Certain of these compounds may mimic all or some of the effects of stimulating the sympathetic system and are called sympathomimetic amines. Their mode of action varies, some such

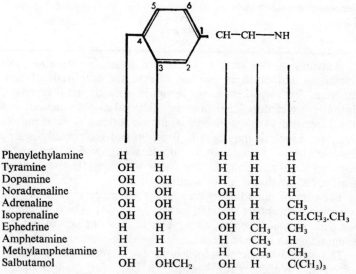

Phenylethylamine	H	H	H	H	H
Tyramine	OH	H	H	H	H
Dopamine	OH	OH	H	H	H
Noradrenaline	OH	OH	OH	H	H
Adrenaline	OH	OH	OH	H	CH_3
Isoprenaline	OH	OH	OH	H	$CH.CH_3.CH_3$
Ephedrine	H	H	OH	CH_3	CH_3
Amphetamine	H	H	H	CH_3	H
Methylamphetamine	H	H	H	CH_3	CH_3
Salbutamol	OH	$OHCH_2$	OH	H	$C(CH_3)_3$

The structure of sympathomimetic amines.

as isoprenaline stimulate the receptors directly though others, such as amphetamine or ephedrine, cause a release of noradrenaline from the storage sites and this then acts on the adrenergic receptors.

The naturally occurring sympathomimetic amines are noradrenaline, adrenaline and dopamine. Ephedrine does not occur in the body but is found in plants of the genus *Ephedra*. The actions of the sympathomimetic amines at first seem very complicated but, in the body, their primary actions of myocardial augmentation, vasodilatation and vasoconstriction provoke compensatory reflexes which produce a varied picture dependent on the drug, the dose and state of the body functions at the time.

Adrenaline, for example, having a predominantly β action produces a net vasodilatation for, though it constricts the blood vessels of the skin, it dilates those of the liver and the skeletal muscle, therefore the total peripheral resistance decreases and the diastolic blood pressure will fall. The direct action of adrenaline on the myocardium will increase rate and force so the cardiac output rises and the systolic blood pressure will increase though due to the fall in diastolic blood pressure, the mean arterial blood pressure remains fairly constant and will not evoke baroceptor reflexes.

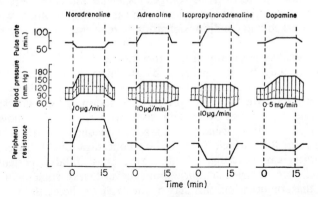

FIG. 7. Cardiovascular effects of infusions of noradrenaline, adrenaline, isopropylnoradrenaline (isoprenaline) and dopamine. (Reproduced from *Brit. med. Bull.* (1963) **19**, 132.)

Infusions were made intravenously during the time indicated by the broken lines. Heart rate is given in beats/min., blood pressure in mm Hg and peripheral resistance in arbitrary units.

Noradrenaline, on the other hand, has a predominantly α action, constricting muscle and liver arterioles and so produces a net vasoconstriction. The total peripheral resistance rises and the mean arterial pressure increases and will evoke a baroceptor response with slowing of the heart. These actions are illustrated in Fig. 7 which should be carefully studied until the reasons for the changes are understood.

Adrenaline

Adrenaline is a racemic compound as it has an asymmetrical carbon atom. The laevo form is some twenty times as potent as the dextro form. It is a weak unstable base, forming salts which are fairly stable in acid solutions but oxidizes rapidly to give a brown colour in alkaline solutions or if exposed to light.

Adrenaline is not active by mouth and has to be given parenterally. It has mainly β actions but some α actions also (Table III). Its effects on the circulation have been discussed above. The metabolic actions increase cell metabolism and liver glycogenolysis to cause hyperglycaemia, glycosuria, release of corticotrophin and increased recovery of fatigued skeletal muscle. There is a constant secretion of adrenaline from the adrenal medulla, which rises markedly in conditions of stress to reinforce local adrenergic activity.

Adrenaline has many uses in therapeutics:

(i) It may be administered by injection to treat asthmatic attacks by its bronchodilator action; to treat acute allergy and anaphylactic attacks; or to prolong the action of local anaesthetics and other drugs by causing vasoconstriction (and so slowing absorption). It is usually given subcutaneously as Adrenaline Injection B.P. which is a 1/1000 concentration. Intravenous injection can be dangerous and even cause fatal hypertensive attacks or ventricular fibrillation; nevertheless some workers feel that, on occasion, this may be the route of choice. Adrenaline is not of much use to raise a low blood pressure and other sympathomimetic amines are preferred for this purpose.

(ii) Adrenaline may be used topically to produce vasoconstriction and to lessen bleeding. It may also be used by aerosol for its bronchodilator action to treat asthmatic attacks.

Noradrenaline

Noradrenaline has mainly α actions, though β actions are also present. Its metabolic function is much less than that of adrenaline and its main task is to act as the neurotransmitter at adrenergic nerve endings.

The major therapeutic use of noradrenaline is to act as a pressor agent in the hypotension of acute circulatory failure. Noradrenaline Injection B.P. is given, well diluted in isotonic saline and administered by slow intravenous infusion, and the dose adjusted to maintain a satisfactory level of blood pressure.

Although noradrenaline causes the blood pressure to rise in acute circulatory failure, its action might be harmful as the vasoconstriction could increase plasma volume loss and cause further deterioration. It might be better to use an isoprenaline infusion to increase cardiac output by a β effect. Dopamine has a similar action to noradrenaline and though far less potent, also dilates the renal vessels which is therapeutically desirable. Other drugs such as metaraminol and mephentermine also have powerful β actions. α adrenergic blocking drugs have also been used in acute circulatory failure though their use is controversial.

Isoprenaline (isoproterenol)

This compound is synthetic and is closely related to noradrenaline. It has practically pure β actions though these are not selective and isoprenaline affects both β_1 and β_2 receptors, (see page 61). It is used therapeutically for its action in relaxing the bronchi (e.g. in asthma) and is given as an aerosol or sublingually. Isoprenaline is not effective orally as it is rapidly inactivated by the gut flora and by catechol-o-methyl transferase (COMT) in the liver. The effects are very rapid in onset though last only briefly. Isoprenaline also maintains the ventricular rate during heart block and may be used as an infusion to treat the acute circulatory failure of myocardial infarction.

Ephedrine

This compound is an alkaloid originally obtained from plants of the genus *Ephedra* but is now synthesized. It is stable in solution, active by mouth and acts by releasing catecholamines from the nerve-ending stores. This mode of action may account for the observation that quickly repeated doses of ephedrine produce less and less effect, a phenomenon known as tachyphylaxis, as perhaps the stores become temporarily depleted.

Ephedrine is not destroyed by amine oxidase and acts as a competitive antagonist of it and so may potentiate the effects of circulating adrenaline and noradrenaline. It has a stimulant effect on the central nervous system. Therapeutically it is used for its bronchodilator action; to decongest the nasal mucosa by topical application; and for its central stimulant action.

Amphetamine (see also page 231)

Amphetamine is synthetic and a racemic base of which the dextro isomer (dexamphetamine) is the more potent. Like ephedrine, it is stable and effective by mouth and acts by release of catecholamines from the nerve store. It causes typical adrenergic effects. It also has a marked central stimulant action which elevates mood, temporarily relieves fatigue and diminishes appetite.

Amphetamine is used for the treatment of depression and anxiety states; as an aid to dieting; and for its analeptic action (page 221). Prolonged use may cause psychic dependence (page 238), various mental symptoms and even frank psychosis.

Metaraminol; mephentermine

These two synthetic sympathomimetic amines have powerful pressor actions which are prolonged as they are not readily inactivated. They may be given intramuscularly or intravenously.

Salbutamol

Previous β-adrenergic drugs (e.g. isoprenaline) act both on the β-receptors of the heart (β_1) and those of the bronchi (β_2). This may cause undesirable increases in heart rate and pulse pressure if they are used to produce bronchodilatation.

Salbutamol has a high degree of selectivity for the β_2-receptors of bronchial smooth muscle and its chronotropic activity is very low. It has a prolonged action of four hours or more when given by inhalation. Salbutamol also has high activity when given orally (cf. isoprenaline) as it is neither destroyed by gut flora enzymes or by COMT in the liver.

Orciprenaline

This resorcinol derivative has both β_1 and β_2 stimulant activity. It is longer acting than isoprenaline and may be used both orally and by inhalation to produce bronchodilatation.

Tyramine

Injection of tyramine causes a strong pressor action due to the release of noradrenaline from the nerve endings. It occurs in many foods such as cheese or yeast extract, but is such a good substrate for MAO that it is rapidly destroyed. If MAO is inhibited (page 232) enough tyramine from the food reaches the systemic circulation to cause severe hypertension.

ADRENERGIC ANTAGONISTS

It has already been stated that catecholamines are liberated from the adrenergic nerve ending and act, after release, upon the adrenergic receptor, and that their actions are terminated mainly by re-uptake into the stores but with some enzymic degradation. Drugs may interfere with this mechanism at several sites either by interfering with release from the stores or by preventing the catecholamines from acting on the effector cell even if released.

Adrenergic neurone blocking drugs (sympatholytic drugs). These drugs interfere with the normal synthesis, release or re-uptake of catecholamines at the nerve ending and have no effect on the adrenergic receptor. Injected sympathomimetic amines, such as noradrenaline, which act directly on the receptor, still have an effect which may be enhanced as one of the usual methods of terminating its action by return to the store may be blocked and so it remains longer on the receptor. Drugs, such as ephedrine, which act by releasing catecholamines from the store, have their actions abolished.

Adrenergic receptor blocking drugs (adrenolytic drugs). These prevent the response of the effector cell to sympathomimetic amines whether released or injected. There are two kinds: those which block α actions and those which block β actions. They act by competitive antagonism and neither alter the adrenergic transmitter substances or affect their release. Circulating adrenaline and noradrenaline are antagonized more readily than the effects of adrenergic nerve stimulation.

Adrenergic Neurone-blocking Drugs

1. *The Rauwolfia alkaloids.* Crude extracts from plants of the genus Rauwolfia have long been used in India for their sedative effect (page 228).

Reserpine is a pure crystalline alkaloid from the plant *R. serpentina.* Others have been purified (rescinnamine, deserpidine) and there are semi-synthetic derivatives (syrosingopine, 10 methoxy-deserpidine).

The hypotension caused by reserpine is probably due to the impairment of adrenergic discharge by the depleted catecholamines of the peripheral nerve stores. This depletion may be the result of reduced uptake rather than active release. Reserpine also depletes the brain of noradrenaline and 5-hydroxytryptamine which may account for the sedation produced (page 228). Claims have been made that derivatives of reserpine such as syrosingopine are less sedative, but the evidence is equivocal.

When reserpine is given in the usual small doses by mouth, its full hypotensive effect may take up to several weeks to develop but if given intramuscularly in large doses its action is swift. The action of reserpine persists long (days to weeks) after administration ceases and the drug has left the body ('hit and run' drug). The major therapeutic use of reserpine is in the treatment of hypertension (page 149), but side effects limits its use. These include bradycardia, diarrhoea, nasal stuffiness, fluid retention and depression. The mental depression has on occasion led to suicide.

2. *Guanethidine.* This drug depletes the catecholamine store and also interferes with the release of transmitter by the nerve impulse. Like reserpine this leads to an impairment of adrenergic nerve discharge and the end result is hypotension, predominantly postural, and due to a decreased cardiac output. Unlike the ganglion-blocking drugs there is no associated parasympathetic block but the effects of circulating sympathomimetic drugs (those which act directly on the adrenergic receptors) will be enhanced.

Guanethidine is used clinically to control hypertension but has a slowly developing action over 4–5 days on oral administration and the effects may persist for several weeks after stopping the drug. On intravenous administration, the blood pressure falls rapidly though there may be an initial rise due apparently to release of noradrenaline from the storage sites. The side effects are mainly those of sympathetic block with a proportionate parasympathetic overactivity. They include postural hypotension, diarrhoea, bradycardia and failure of ejaculation.

3. *Bethanidine*. This drug has essentially the same effects as guanethidine though these are quicker of onset. On oral administration the effect is maximum in 4–5 hours and subsides by 12 hours. The side effects are similar to guanethidine but it gives less diarrhoea.

4. *Debrisoquine*. This adrenergic neurone blocking drug acts at the neuro-effector junction, though unlike guanethidine it does not deplete tissue stores of noradrenaline. It produces a fall in blood pressure in 2–4 hours lasting 9–24 hours. The side effects are similar to bethanidine.

5. *Guanoxan*. This drug blocks the release of noradrenaline from the adrenergic neurone and depletes the stores. It also has α adrenergic receptor blocking action. Its side effects are similar to those of guanethidine but also include the possibility of impaired liver function.

6. *α-Methyldopa*. This drug inhibits the action of dopa decarboxylase which decarboxylates dopa to dopamine (Table II). It was thought that the hypotensive action of methyldopa was due to the inhibition of noradrenaline synthesis with consequent depletion of the nerve ending store. Recent evidence is not in agreement with this though some little depletion may occur. It may be that methyldopa also acts as a substrate to dopa decarboxylase to form α-methyl dopamine and α-methyl noradrenaline which displace noradrenaline from the nerve stores. These false transmitters have a weaker pressor action than the normal transmitters and as they are not destroyed by MAO, they are persistent in the stores. Recently, however, doubt has been cast on this hypothesis and it may be that a central action is involved. α methyldopa readily passes the blood–brain barrier and could there be converted to α methyldopamine and α methylnoradrenaline which *could* stimulate central α adrenoceptors connected to inhibitory

pathways and produce a reduction of sympathetic outflow (see clonidine, page 151).

Methyldopa also interferes with the synthesis of 5-hydroxy-tryptamine (serotonin) by inhibiting the decarboxylation of 5-hydroxytryptophan (which is probably also due to dopa decar-boxylase). This could lead to a fall in the amount of 5-hydroxy-tryptamine in the brain and may play a role in the sedative action seen with methyldopa. Other side effects include depression, dreams and hallucinations. Tolerance may become a problem when methyldopa is used in the treatment of hypertension.

7. *Guanoclor*. This drug inhibits the action of dopamine oxi-dase, which catalyses the formation of noradrenaline from dopa-mine. Although used in the treatment of hypertension, it is difficult to get steady falls of blood pressure.

8. *Monoamine oxidase inhibitors*. Drugs such as pargyline inhibit the enzyme monoamine oxidase (MAO) which catalyses part of the metabolic degradation of the catecholamines. Apart from their antidepressant action (page 232), they also produce hypotension by adrenergic neurone block. It may seem strange that a substance inhibiting the enzyme which breaks down noradrenaline should produce hypotension and not hypertension. However, it is likely that the catecholamines are degraded by other routes when the MAO pathway is blocked and these meta-bolites have less pressor action than normal.

Monoamine oxidase inhibitors have the great disadvantage of numerous food and drug interactions. Foods such as cheese, or yeast extract contain a large amount of tyramine (page 67) which is normally rapidly destroyed by MAO but if the enzyme is inhibited, the excess tyramine causes noradrenaline release which may provoke dangerous rises in blood pressure.

9. *Cocaine*. This drug potentiates adrenergic mechanisms as well as being a local anaesthetic (page 242). The potentiation is probably caused by the prevention of re-uptake of noradrenaline by the stores, which then remains longer in contact with the receptors. Cocaine also inhibits monoamine oxidase and has a stimulant action on the nervous system which accounts for its addictive nature. Its effect on the eye when instilled into the con-junctival sac is discussed on page 77.

Adrenergic Receptor-blocking Drugs

1. α-Adrenergic receptor-blocking drugs

These drugs prevent stimulation of the α-adrenergic receptor by sympathomimetic substances whether released or injected.

(i) *Imidazoline derivatives*. Tolazoline and phentolamine have a brief and moderately powerful α-blocking action. They also have some sympathomimetic effects such as tachycardia and coronary vasodilatation. There are also some parasympathomimetic and histamine-like actions such as nausea, vomiting, diarrhoea. Clonidine is also an imidazoline derivative but is more active at central receptors and is used to treat hypertension (page 152) and migraine.

(ii) *β-Haloalkylamines*. Dibenamine and phenoxybenzamine have a specific and prolonged α-blocking action. Phenoxybenzamine can be given by mouth or injection and the effects last 2–4 days.

(iii) *Ergot alkaloids*. These are discussed in detail on page 95. The amino acid alkaloids such as ergotoxine and ergotamine are powerful smooth muscle stimulants as well as α-adrenergic blockers. The amine alkaloids such as ergometrine have no α-blocking action but are powerful oxytocics.

(iv) *Chlorpromazine and other phenothiazine derivatives*. These have a minor α-adrenergic blocking action (page 226).

(v) *Thymoxamine*. This α-receptor blocking drug has few other actions but has a short half life and is unreliably absorbed by mouth.

Therapeutic indications for α-receptor block

(i) *Hypertension*. Most α-receptor blocking drugs are of little use in the treatment of hypertension as they produce a postural hypotension which is often not predictable even when given in high dose. The hypotension is due to the abolition of peripheral vasoconstriction and the lowering of the total peripheral resistance. It is offset by a compensatory tachycardia which is a β-response and is not affected.

(ii) *Phaeochromocytoma*. Blockade of α-receptors is of value to prevent the hypertensive episodes characteristic of this adrenal medulla tumour. β-blockade is also necessary.

(iii) *Shock.* α-Receptor blocking drugs have been used in the treatment of acute hypotensive states to produce vasodilatation to encourage blood flow to the vital organs.

(iv) *Peripheral vascular disease.* α-Blocking drugs are sometimes used especially where the peripheral ischaemia is due to spasm rather than organic disease. Their value is disputed as they tend to increase skin rather than muscle blood flow.

2. β-adrenergic receptor blocking drugs

These drugs prevent the β-agonist actions of compounds like isoprenaline by competitive antagonism and in general are very similar structurally. Dichloroisoprenaline (DCI) was the first effective member of the group but its intrinsic sympathomimetic (i.e. agonist) activity before block occurred make it unsuitable for therapeutic use. Recent developments have produced drugs like practolol with some selectivity in the β-receptor they block (i.e. β_1 or β_2, see page 61) though this selectivity tends to be relative rather than absolute and is dose dependent.

(i) *Propranolol.* Propranolol is a racemic mixture and the L-isomer blocks both β_1 and β_2 receptors whereas both the L- and D-isomer possess local anaesthetic (quinidine-like, membrane stabilizing) actions. It has little intrinsic sympathomimetic actions.

This non-selective β-blockade results in a fall in heart rate, cardiac output, systolic blood pressure and left ventricular work especially in the erect position and in the response to exercise. It can precipitate heart failure as the function of a failing heart may be critically dependent on the sympathetic drive. As sympathetically mediated bronchodilatation will be blocked by propranolol, care must be taken with asthmatic patients as sympathetic bronchodilators will no longer be effective.

(ii) *Practolol.* This drug has a selective (dose-dependent) action on β_1 receptors (i.e. those affecting the heart, see page 61) in doses not affecting the β_2 receptors. It also has a transient sympathomimetic action but no local anaesthetic activity. Practolol has recently been associated with diminished tear secretion, sclerosing peritonitis, deafness and psoriaform rashes. The relevance of this to other β blockers is uncertain.

(iii) *Oxprenolol*. Like propranolol, this drug is non-selective and blocks both β_1 and β_2 receptors. It has mild initial sympathomimetic activity.

Therapeutic indications for β-receptor block

(i) *Angina pectoris* (see page 148). The reduction in cardiac work produced by the β-blocking drugs may be of value.

(ii) *Arrhythmias*. Drugs like propranolol may be of use in the treatment of various cardiac arrhythmias though this seems to be due to their β-receptor blocking properties and not their local anaesthetic or quinidine-like action (page 143).

(iii) *Hypertension*. β-receptor blocking drugs may be of use in the treatment of hypertension either alone or in combination with other drugs. The fall in blood pressure they produce is probably due to the fall in cardiac output.

(iv) *Anxiety* (see page 230). Excessive sympathetic effects such as tachycardia, 'palpitations' and sweating are often characteristic of anxiety states and may be controlled by the use of β-receptor blocking drugs.

(v) *Hyperthyroidism* (see page 127).

AUTONOMIC DRUGS ON THE EYE

The action of autonomic drugs on the eye is important as an illustration of their actions and for their therapeutic use. Drugs may be applied to the conjunctiva to pass into the eyeball and have very localized effects. To understand these, it is necessary to revise briefly the innervation of the eye; the mechanics of focusing the lens and altering the diameter of the pupil.

1. The Autonomic Innervation of the Eye

(a) Parasympathetic supply

The preganglionic neurones originate in the oculomotor nucleus and the axons travel in the oculomotor nerve to the ciliary ganglion. The axons of the post-ganglionic neurones then travel in the short ciliary nerves to the ciliary muscle and constrictor muscle of the iris. When the ciliary muscle relaxes, the suspensory ligament (zonule) tightens by elastic recoil and flattens the lens to focus it for distant vision. Stimulation of the

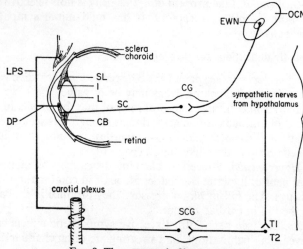

FIG. 8. The autonomic fibres to the eye.

OCN   oculomotor nucleus
EWN   Edinger–Westphal nucleus
CG   ciliary ganglion
SCG   superior cervical ganglion
T1   first segment of the thoracic spinal cord
T2   second segment of the thoracic spinal cord
DP   sympathetic nerve to dilator pupillae
LPS   sympathetic nerve to levator palpebrae superioris
SL   suspensory ligaments of the lens
L   lens
I   iris
CB   ciliary body
CP   constrictor pupillae
SC   parasympathetic fibres (short ciliary nerves) to ciliary body and constrictor pupillae.

parasympathetic causes constriction of the pupil (miosis) and accommodation for near vision as the ciliary muscle contracts and releases the tension on the suspensory ligament thus changing the curvature and focus of the lens.

(b) Sympathetic supply

The preganglionic neurones originate in the upper thoracic segments and their axons ascend the sympathetic chain to the superior cervical ganglion. The axons of the post-ganglionic neurone then travel via the carotid plexus and the long ciliary nerves to the dilator muscle of the iris, the smooth muscle of levator palpebrae superioris and the blood vessels of the retina, orbit and conjunctiva. In lower animals (e.g. cat) they supply the nictitating membrane. Stimulation of the sympathetic nerves causes pupillary dilatation (mydriasis), vasoconstriction, and elevation of the upper lid.

2. The Aqueous Humour

This is in the anterior chamber of the eye and is continuously produced by the ciliary bodies to escape via the sinus venosus sclerae (Canal of Schlemm) at the irido-corneal (filtration) angle. If this escape is impeded, the intraocular pressure rises as the secretion of fluid continues and may give rise to the clinical condition of glaucoma. The canal may be blocked due to the hardening and narrowing consequent on age or by mechanical pressure from a widely dilated iris.

3. The Local Use of Drugs in the Eye

Drugs are instilled into the conjunctival sac for their local effect on the eye and are discussed below. Their systemic effects are mentioned elsewhere.

(a) Parasympathomimetic drugs

These produce effects similar to stimulation of the oculomotor nerve (constriction of the pupil and eye focused for near vision), which also occurs if the oculomotor centre is stimulated (e.g. by morphine) or if the inhibitory action of the higher centres is lessened by sleep or anaesthetics.

Physostigmine (page 48) potentiates the muscarine-like actions of acetylcholine by antagonism of cholinesterases to cause miosis, ciliary spasm and fixing of the lens for near vision. The intraocular pressure may fall due to the opening out of the filtration angle by the stretched iris which facilitates reabsorption of the aqueous. Accommodation may return to normal in 3 hours but the miosis starts in a few minutes, is maximal in 30 minutes and may not wear off for several days. Physostigmine is used to treat glaucoma or to counteract the effect of mydriatics. Drugs with similar effects are ecothiopate (a long-acting cholinesterase) and pilocarpine (page 47), an alkaloid which stimulates cholinergic receptors.

(b) Drugs blocking the muscarine-like actions of acetylcholine

Atropine. This drug antagonizes the muscarine-like actions of acetylcholine and so will paralyse the ciliaris and the constrictor pupillae to give dilatation of the pupil (mydriasis) due to unopposed action of the dilator, paralysis of accommodation (cycloplegia) with fixation of the lens for far vision. The paralysis of the constrictor pupillae causes loss of the light reflex. A 1% solution of atropine instilled into the conjunctival sac produces maximal dilatation of the pupil in about 30–60 minutes for 7–10 days. More than an hour may be necessary for the paralysis of accommodation which persists for 3–5 days. Mydriatics such as atropine are used to dilate the pupil to facilitate ophthalmological examination. In inflammation of the iris, they will rest the eye and the dilatation of the pupil will keep the iris away from the lens and prevent adhesions. The persistent mydriasis may cause blockage of the filtration angle and provoke glaucoma in susceptible persons.

Homatropine (page 51) acts similarly to atropine but is less potent, with a quicker onset of action which lasts for 12–24 hours, but may be unreliable in children. *Hyoscine* (page 51) may also be used for its antimuscarine-like actions and has an intermediate duration of effect. *Lachesine* may be used in people sensitive to other atropine-like drugs. *Cyclopentolate* has a mydriatic action of about 6–12 hours.

(c) Sympathomimetic drugs

These cause dilatation of the pupil by stimulation of dilator pupillae so that the light reflex will still be present as constrictor pupillae is not affected (cf. atropine). They will also cause pallor of the sclera due to vasoconstriction and retraction of the upper eye lid due to stimulation of adrenergically innervated smooth muscle in levator palpebrae superioris.

Adrenaline and phenylephrine dilate the pupil though have

little effect on accommodation. The intraocular pressure may fall, perhaps by reducing the formation of aqueous. Cocaine also stimulates adrenergic mechanisms (page 70) to give similar effects. It is also a local anaesthetic and will abolish the corneal reflex though high doses may produce cycloplegia.

(d) Drugs blocking sympathetic activity in the eye

Drugs like guanethidine (page 68) paralyse dilator pupillae and leave the constrictor pupillae unopposed to produce a small pupil. They may also produce ptosis (a drooping of the upper eyelid) and will antagonize the actions of sympathomimetic drugs.

REFERENCES

Goodman, L. S. & Gilman, A. (1975) *The Pharmacological Basis of Therapeutics*, 5th edn. Baillière Tindall: London, New York: Macmillan.

Robson, J. M. & Stacey, R. S. (eds.) (1968) *Recent Advances in Pharmacology*, 4th edn. pp. 135–154, 155–177, 178–184. London: Churchill.

Catecholamines (1973) *British Medical Bulletin*, **29** (2).

8   Voluntary Muscle and the Neuromuscular Junction

A motor nerve fibre from a spinal motor neurone branches to supply as many as 5 to 300 muscle fibres, the whole forming a motor unit. There is no anatomical continuity between the nerve terminal and the muscle fibre but there is very close and intimate contact with the nerve terminal lying in grooves indenting a specialized area of the muscle fibre, the motor end plate (post-synaptic membrane) (Fig. 9).

Transmission of the nerve impulse across the synaptic gap is by a nicotine-like action of acetylcholine which is present in little vesicles in the nerve ending. It is released into the synaptic gap to act on the motor end plate which is very sensitive to it and becomes permeable to small cations like Na^+ and K^+ to give first a simple depolarization which, on reaching a threshold value, is propagated as a muscle action potential and a contraction initiated. There is a constant release of small amounts of acetylcholine causing miniature end plate potentials (mepp) which summate when the nerve impulse reaches the terminals to give the effective end plate potential (eepp). The release of acetylcholine from the vesicles depends on the calcium concentration which rises during activity and probably alters the vesicles so that they spill their contents into the synaptic gap. The released acetylcholine is quickly destroyed by cholinesterases which are present mainly on the surface of the motor end plate in palisade cells. The motor end plate and the muscle fibre rapidly repolarize to become ready for the next nerve impulse.

The acetylcholine is synthesized in the body of the nerve cell by the acetylation of choline by choline acetyltransferase and acetyl

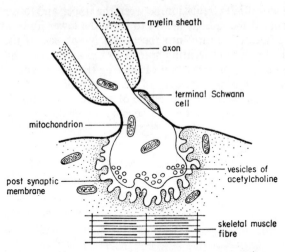

myelin sheath

axon

terminal Schwann cell

mitochondrion

post synaptic membrane

vesicles of acetylcholine

skeletal muscle fibre

FIG. 9. Diagram of the skeletal neuromuscular junction.

coenzyme A, and is stored in the vesicles which stream down the axon and accumulate in the synaptic region.

NEUROMUSCULAR BLOCKING DRUGS

It is possible to block the transmission of the nerve impulse across the neuromuscular junction by drugs that do not affect either the conduction of the nerve impulse along the motor nerve or the contractile power of the muscle fibre. These drugs are called neuromuscular blocking drugs or muscle relaxants. The muscle will no longer respond to nerve (or indirect) stimulation) but will respond to muscle (or direct stimulation).

The classic neuromuscular blocking drug is curare and the action of this drug was admirably shown by Claude Bernard in 1856. In a series of very simple experiments he demonstrated that the action of curare was not in the nerve trunk or muscle fibre but at their junction and that the sensory and central components of the reflex arc were unimpaired. This reflex arc may be taken in its simplest form to consist of three parts, a sensory or receptor part, the central nervous part, and the motor or effector part (Fig. 10). Bernard ligated the lumbar region of a

frog to cut off all circulation between the upper and lower halves
but excluded the lumbar nerves to leave the lower limbs innervated. He injected curare into the dorsal lymph sac of the upper
half; the ligature preventing spread to the lower half and found
that stimulation of either half of the frog (i.e. the receptor part of
the reflex arc) gave movement of the lower half only (the effector
part). This showed that the action of curare is peripheral, on the
motor nerve, and not on the sensory or central limbs of the
reflex arc.

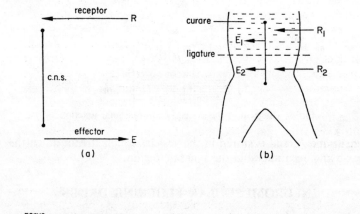

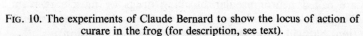

Fig. 10. The experiments of Claude Bernard to show the locus of action of
curare in the frog (for description, see text).
(a) The reflex arc
(b) Frog with lumbar ligature
(c) The isolated sciatic-gastrocnemius preparation

A second series of experiments by Bernard used the isolated
sciatic-gastrocnemius preparation of the frog in which the nerve
and muscle were immersed separately in curare solution. The
immersed muscle responded only to direct stimulation and not
to stimulation via the nerve. When the nerve only was immersed
there was a muscle response to both direct and indirect stimula-

tion. This showed that the action of curare must be at the junction
of the nerve and the muscle.

Production of Neuromuscular Block

It is possible to produce neuromuscular block by reducing the
output of transmitter from the nerve ending with drugs such as
hemicholinium or local anaesthetics; by ion changes such as a fall
in calcium concentration; or by diphtheria and botulinus toxins.

Drugs which block the motor end plate are more important
in clinical practice and are used mainly to provide muscle relaxation in operative surgery but sometimes also as a life-saving
measure to prevent convulsions in such disorders as tetanus and
during electro-convulsive therapy. Although they produce relaxation and abolish muscle reflexes, the muscle relaxants have no effect
on consciousness or the appreciation of pain, so hypnotic and
analgesic drugs must be given also during surgical operations.

The mode of action of block at the motor end plate is of two
main kinds: the curare-like ('anti-depolarizing or competitive')
block and the depolarizing (or desensitization) block. There is also
a dual or mixed block with depolarizing and curare-like components.

Curare-like or competitive block. The drug competes with
acetylcholine for the motor end plate receptors to prevent depolarization (i.e. antidepolarizing block). This antagonism is competitive (page 22 and Fig. 1) so if the concentration of acetylcholine
is raised (e.g. by the use of anticholinesterases), the block may be
wholly or partially overcome. The block is analogous to that
produced by atropine at the muscarine sites of action of acetylcholine.

Depolarization or densitization block. The drug depolarizes
the motor end plate in a similar fashion to acetylcholine, but
recovery is slow to occur. As the muscle becomes relaxed, perhaps
after a few induced contractions, depolarization alone does not
occur for otherwise the muscle would remain contracted. The
motor end plate depolarizes and then becomes electrically inexcit-
able (desensitization block) though the muscle itself repolarizes,
relaxes and can be stimulated directly though not via the nerve.
In depolarization block, if the acetylcholine concentration is
allowed to build up (e.g. by the use of anticholinesterase), then,

unlike competitive block, depolarization block is not reversed and may worsen as the excessive acetylcholine produces even more depolarization.

Individual Muscle Relaxants

1. *Tubocurarine*. This drug is a pure alkaloid extracted from curare. It is a quaternary ammonium compound (a bis-onium) and is usually given as the dextro-isomer as the laevo-isomer is much less potent. Like all quaternary ammoniums, it is poorly absorbed from the gut and must be given intravenously. Curare itself is used as an arrow poison by South American Indians, and the poor absorption from the gut enables animals that have been poisoned by curare to be eaten safely. Tubocurarine is evenly distributed in the plasma and is rapidly cleared either in the urine as the unchanged drug or metabolized.

On intravenous administration, tubocurarine causes a flaccid paralysis with no initial stimulation, which is maximal in four minutes and lasts about half an hour. The paralysis begins in the eyes and small muscles of the hands and spreads to the face, limbs, trunk and intercostal muscles and finally to the diaphragm. Its mode of action by competitive block and the ready reversibility by anticholinesterases has already been discussed. Tubocurarine also has some ganglionic blocking action, is potentiated by ether and causes some histamine release.

2. *Gallamine triethiodide*. This is a synthetic compound and, like tubocurarine, is a quaternary ammonium. It has a similar action to tubocurarine, but also has an atropine-like action so the heart rate and blood pressure may rise due to vagal antagonism. It has no ganglion-blocking or histamine-releasing effect but is potentiated by ether. On a weight basis it is one-fifth as potent as tubocurarine and has a slightly shorter action.

3. *Decamethonium*. This drug is a member of the bis-quaternary ammonium series (page 55) and has ten methylene groups in the connecting chain, so neuromuscular-blocking properties predominate. The block is of the depolarization type. Decamethonium also has very weak histamine-releasing properties and very weak anti-true cholinesterase actions. It is mainly excreted unchanged via the urine.

4. *Suxamethonium* (*succinycholine*). This drug is in effect two

molecules of acetylcholine joined and produces a brief depolarization block beginning in less than a minute and lasting for 5–10 minutes.

It is hydrolysed by pseudocholinesterases to choline and succinyl monocholine. Succinyl monocholine has very weak blocking activity and is further hydrolysed to succinic acid and choline. Some people are naturally deficient in pseudocholinesterases and the action of suxamethonium may then be very prolonged and can cause arrest of respiration (suxamethonium apnoea). Pseudocholinesterases may also be inhibited by a low body temperature or by anticholinesterases to give this picture of prolonged suxamethonium action.

The depolarizing action of suxamethonium may cause initial muscle fasciculations which could be the cause of postoperative deep muscle pain felt by some patients.

5. *Pancuronium*. This synthetic muscle relaxant releases less histamine than tubocurarine.

The chemical structure of neuromuscular blocking drugs

The primary requirement of a neuromuscular blocking drug is a strongly basic centre capable of permanent existence as a positively charged ion, the onium centre. This centre is possessed by quaternary ammonium compounds and analogues such as sulphonium, phosphonium, arsonium and stibonium radicals. This suggests that the essential reaction is an ionic one involving a complementary anionic centre on the receptor molecule. The two quaternary ammonium groups in tubocurarine, decamethonium and suxamethonium are each separated by 15 Å though the intervening groups are different. This suggests that the interquaternary distance is concerned with the primary two point attachment to the receptor molecule after which secondary groups determine the type of physiological response. Much remains to be learnt before definite theories emerge on these structure-effect relationships.

Evaluation of the neuromuscular blocking drugs

These may be evaluated in the laboratory either in the whole animal or on isolated preparations. Various methods are used in the whole animal from the production of paralysis in frogs and tadpoles to the reduction of handgrip or respiratory volume in man. Intravenous tubocurarine in the chicken produces a flaccid paralysis whereas decamethonium and other depolarizing drugs cause a spastic paralysis thus allowing a quick distinction between them. Isolated preparations include the various nerve muscle preparations such as the sciatic-gastrocnemius of the frog; the quadriceps of the cat, and the phrenic nerve-diaphragm of the rat or kitten.

STIMULANTS OF SKELETAL MUSCLE

Skeletal muscle may be stimulated by the application of acetylcholine either to the endplate itself or injected into the artery supplying the muscle. By all other routes acetylcholine is quickly destroyed and ineffective. More stable esters such as carbachol cause contractions of skeletal muscle but have a predominant muscarine-like action which makes them unsuitable for therapeutic use.

Anticholinesterases (page 47) will prolong the nicotine-like action of acetylcholine at the motor end plate though physostigmine and the organophosphorus compounds have muscarinelike actions which also makes them therapeutically unsuitable. Neostigmine and pyridostigmine have a more marked nicotinelike action as well as a direct stimulant effect on skeletal muscle which lasts for several hours.

Myasthenia gravis. This pathological condition is characterized by extreme muscle weakness as acetylcholine does not exert its normal stimulant action at the motor end plate. Anticholinesterases may relieve the condition and both neostigmine and pyridostigmine are used for this purpose. Edrophonium may be used in the diagnosis of myasthenia gravis and to assess the probable beneficial effects of anticholinesterases. Its actions are brief and include a direct nicotine-like effect.

REFERENCES

Bovet, D., Bovet-Nitti, F. & Marinini Bettolo, G. B. (1959) *Curare and Curare-like Agents.* Amsterdam: Elsevier.

Bowman, W. (1962) Mechanisms of neuromuscular blockade. In *Progress in Medical Chemistry*, **2**, 43. Ellis, G. P. & West, G. B. (eds.). London: Butterworth.

Bryn Jones, K. (1964) *Curare, its History and Usage*. London: Pitman Medical.

Stenlake, J. B. (1963) Some chemical aspects of neuromuscular block. In *Progress in Medicinal Chemistry*, **3**, 1. Ellis, G. P. & West, G. B. (eds.). London: Butterworth.

9   Smooth Muscle

The compounds considered in this chapter are a heterogeneous group with widely differing structures and pharmacological activity. They act especially on the smooth muscle of the gut, blood vessels and bronchi. Some of them are of especial interest as they occur in the body, but have functions that are by no means understood. Some of these substances, such as 5-hydroxytryptamine, angiotensin I, bradykinin and the prostaglandins, rapidly disappear in the pulmonary circulation and hence are unlikely to reach the arterial circulation unless the lungs are overwhelmed, as may happen in some disease states. They probably act at the site of release as local hormones or tissue hormones though some prefer the term autacoid (Gk. *autos*, self; *akos*, medicinal agent).

HISTAMINE

The function of histamine is still much a mystery, though it plays a part in many physiological processes and is distributed through the animal and plant kingdoms. In mammals it occurs especially in the mast cells of the skin, lungs and intestinal mucosa as intracellular particles, perhaps in association with heparin. Histamine turnover in the mast cells is extremely slow (half-life 50 days) but histamine is also found in other tissues, e.g. the brain and stomach in which the synthesis and turnover is much more rapid. Histamine is also found in many plant and insect venoms.

Chemically, histamine is very stable and is formed by the intracellular decarboxylation of histidine, though some is formed in the gut by bacterial action but is not much absorbed, and histamine by mouth produces no pharmacological effects.

Only a very small percentage (1%) appears in the urine unchanged and the rest is metabolized. Some undergoes oxidative deamination by histaminase (diamine oxidase); more than 50% is methylated; some is acetylated, and some inactivated by tissue binding.

The Actions of Histamine

These are especially marked on the vascular system, smooth muscle and exocrine glands. It seems likely that there are at least 2 types of histamine receptor. The H_2-receptor responsible for the effects on gastric secretion (and some of those on blood pressure) and the H_1-receptor responsible for the other effects.

1. *The cardiovascular system.* Histamine dilates the capillaries especially of the face and upper body in man (the blush area) and increases their permeability to plasma proteins. The actions of histamine on the arterioles is species dependent; it causes vasoconstriction and a consequent rise in blood pressure in rats and rabbits but vasodilatation and a fall in blood pressure in dog and man. This vasodilatation causes stretching of pain receptors in the dura matter to give the characteristic histamine headache.

Intradermal injection of histamine causes the classic Triple Response of red line, flare, and weal. The red line is due to the dilatation of the capillaries and the surrounding flare is due to arteriolar dilation caused by an axon reflex. The weal is due to the increase in permeability to plasma proteins which allows them to escape to the extracellular space, thus reducing the osmotic gradient and allowing fluid to leak out also.

2. *Other smooth muscle.* Histamine has a marked bronchoconstrictor effect and stimulates most other smooth muscle.

3. *Exocrine glands.* Histamine stimulates most glands. It will release noradrenaline and adrenaline from the adrenal gland but this is insignificant save in phaeochromocytoma which is a tumour of the adrenal medulla and may be provoked by histamine to release large amounts of noradrenaline and adrenaline to cause dangerous rises in blood pressure.

Histamine is a direct secretogogue on the oxyntic glands, and this action is not antagonized by the antihistamine of the H_1-receptor blocking type (see page 89).

The physiological role of histamine

This is not precisely known. It exists in the body as combined histamine which is released only by cellular destruction; as labile histamine which is released by physical and chemical stimuli and as free histamine in very small amounts.

Histamine may play a part in gastric secretion with the hormone gastrin. It may play a part as a transmitter in the central nervous system. It may also play a part in inflammatory processes, tissue growth and repair and in antibody–antigen reactions.

The liberation of histamine is probably the cause of a number of toxic effects in man and any process involving mechanical, thermal or radiant damage will cause its release. Many drugs also cause histamine release; they include tubocurarine, morphine, pethidine, some antihistamines and some chemotherapeutic agents.

Histamine and allergy

Histamine is released in many allergic states due to antigen-antibody reactions, and the injection of histamine reproduces many of the allergic or anaphylactic symptoms such as the weal of urticaria, bronchoconstriction and hypotension. It is not easy to understand why antihistamines so readily relieve the symptoms of some allergic states such as urticaria but not others such as bronchial asthma. It may be that other substances such as 5-hydroxytryptamine are liberated or perhaps in some cases the histamine is liberated and acts intracellularly (intrinsic histamine) and the antihistamines are unable to reach the site. In some other cases, perhaps, histamine is liberated and has to diffuse to other sites such as blood vessels before acting (extrinsic histamine) and the antihistamines are then able to compete for the histaminergic receptors.

Therapeutic uses of histamine. These are few, but it is used diagnostically in the augmented histamine test of gastric secretion but has recently been replaced by pentagastrin (page 245).

Ametazole. This is a histamine analogue with marked gastric stimulant actions, though with much less prominent other histamine-like effects. It may be given parenterally or by mouth.

ANTIHISTAMINES

It is possible to antagonize the actions of histamine in several ways. One could accelerate the destruction of histamine by the use of the enzyme histaminase but this is not yet practical. Adrenal steroids (page 105) will suppress the effects of antigen–antibody reactions with which histamine is involved (see also disodium cromoglycate, page 95). It is possible to give a drug with the opposite actions to those of histamine acting on non-histamine receptors (e.g. adrenaline) and this may be called non-specific or physiological antagonism.

The actions of histamine may also be antagonized by the use of competitive antagonists (page 22), which because of mass action considerations occupy the receptors that histamine would normally occupy and thus prevent triggering of the usual response. These are known as the antihistamines, and their basic structure includes the group $-CH_2.CH_2.N=$ and as this forms part of the structure of histamine, it is undoubtedly concerned in the agonist–antagonist interactions. The grouping $-CH_2.CH_2.N=$ is also possessed by a variety of compounds not usually classified as antihistamines but which have appreciable antihistamine properties. These include local anaesthetics (e.g. procaine); anti-arrhythmic drugs (e.g. quinidine); tranquillizers (e.g. chlorpromazine); β-haloalkylamine adrenergic blocking drugs (e.g. phenoxybenzamine); and some ganglion blockers.

Antihistamines as a group are readily absorbed by all routes and are usually given by mouth, intramuscularly, or intravenously if speed is necessary. Topical use is to be avoided as it can cause sensitivity reactions. The antihistamines are metabolized mainly in the liver by histaminase and excreted into the urine.

Their actions are many and can be divided into the antihistamine effects and other effects, though the latter are often the reason why the drugs are given.

1. Antihistamine effects

The competitive antihistamines effectively antagonize the actions of injected histamine on smooth muscle H_1-receptors but may not always prevent similar effects occurring in the body which are due to allergic causes. Asthmatic bronchoconstriction, for example, is more or less unaffected by antihistamines whereas broncho· constriction provoked by injected histamine is readily prevented- It may be that endogenous histamine is not easily reached by the competitive antagonist or in allergic states other substances are concerned, such as 5-hydroxytryptamine and Slow Reacting Substance (SRS), which are not so readily antagonized.

The stimulant action of histamine on gastric acid output (H_2-receptors) is not blocked by antihistamine (but see burimamide) and this is made use of in the histamine test meal when the unwanted effects of histamine are suppressed without affecting acid production. The failure of histamine to provoke the output of acid from the stomach (histamine fast achlorhydria) is of diagnostic significance in pernicious anaemia. Recently, investigations have begun into the effects of burimamide. This substance, unlike other antihistamines, blocks the H_2 receptors and so the stimulant effect of histamine on gastric acid output is prevented.

Antihistamines do diminish the effect of histamine on other exocrine glands such as the salivary and nasolacrimal glands.

2. Other effects of antihistamines

(i) *The central nervous system.* Antihistamines are normally sedative but can cause excitement especially in overdose. They are of use in the relief of motion sickness, in vomiting of early pregnancy (page 249) and to lessen the rigidity and tremor of Parkinsonism. The sedation can be troublesome (e.g. car driving) and occurs more frequently with some types such as diphenhydramine.

(ii) *Local analgesic and cardiodepressant actions.* Many antihistamines are quite potent local analgesics and this, together with quinidine-like and cardiodepressant actions, makes them of some use in arrhythmias.

(iii) *Autonomic effects.* Antihistamines are not entirely specific in their antagonism to histamine and in higher concentrations may antagonize acetylcholine. This atropine-like action can cause a dry mouth and suppress nasopharyngeal secretions. Parasympathomimetic actions on the gut may account for the occasional diarrhoea seen with the antihistamines. There may also be sympathomimetic effects.

(iv) *Miscellaneous actions* Some antihistamines may actually cause histamine release and some (e.g. cyproheptadine) may have an anti-5-hydroxytryptamine action. Hypersensitivity and other allergic reactions can occur especially with topical use, and this sensitivity can spread to all types of antihistamines and even to other classes of drugs such as analgesics and antimicrobials. It is difficult to justify topical use.

In acute poisoning with antihistamines, the signs are especially those of central nervous involvement and resemble atropine poisoning. The treatment is symptomatic.

Antihistamines are synergistic with some central nervous depressants such as ethyl alcohol, tranquillizers and monoamine oxidase inhibitors and there may be serious effects if combined therapy is used. Antihistamines occasionally cause other reactions such as dizziness, tinnitus, tremor, diplopia, incoordination and insomnia. Teratogenicity is always a possibility in early pregnancy.

Preparations of antihistamines

Antihistamines vary little in their potency as antagonists of histamine but do vary in chemical type, dosage, duration of action and side effects. They may be grouped as follows:

(i) *Ethanolamines*, e.g. diphenhydramine. These have marked atropine-like and sedative effects but a low incidence of alimentary effects. Their actions last for 4–6 hours.

(ii) *Ethylenediamines*, e.g. mepyramine. These have no marked central nervous effects but can cause nausea and vomiting. Their actions last for 4–6 hours.

(iii) *Propylamines*, e.g. chlorpheniramine. These are very active antihistamines and not prone to cause other effects. Their actions last for 4–6 hours.

(iv) *Piperazines*, e.g. chlorcyclizine. These are especially useful in motion sickness and have actions lasting 8–12 hours.

(v) *Phenothiazines*, e.g. promethazine. These are very similar in structure to the tranquillizer chlorpromazine. They are very sedative and long acting, with a duration of action of 12–24 hours.

(vi) *Various*. This group includes antihistamines such as cyproheptadine, which has an anti-5-hydroxytryptamine action and phenindamine which has a central nervous stimulant action.

5-HYDROXYTRYPTAMINE

5-Hydroxytryptamine (5-HT, serotonin) is distributed throughout the animal and plant kingdoms. It is formed from the amino acid tryptophan which is first hydroxylated to 5-hydroxytryptophan and then decarboxylated to 5-hydroxytryptamine by an enzyme closely related to dopa decarboxylase (see methyldopa, page 69). The major site of inactivation of 5-HT is in the lungs, primarily by an uptake and storage process; enzymic degradation by amine oxidases also occurs.

It is a stimulant of smooth muscle and the heart but has a very variable action due to compensatory reflexes. Injection in man gives overbreathing due to respiratory stimulation accompanied by tachycardia and vasoconstriction. There is also a reduction in urine flow. 5-HT strongly stimulates sensory nerve endings to cause marked pain and is found in various plant and insect venoms.

The physiological function of 5-HT is not known. In man it is found mainly in the intestines in the cells of the enterochromaffin (argentaffin) system and in the brain and platelets. It may be concerned with the local control of peristalsis and may be a neurohumoral transmitter in the central nervous system, though the evidence for this is not conclusive. Deranged 5-HT metabolism has been implicated in schizophrenia and other mental disorders.

5-HT increases capillary permeability and causes local oedema and may be concerned in anaphylactic and allergic reactions in some species such as rats, mice and hamsters, though is probably not important in man.

5-*Hydroxytryptamine antagonists*. The actions of 5-HT can be antagonized in several ways. Drugs may be given which exert the opposite effects (physiological antagonists). Drugs may also antagonize the action of 5-HT indirectly by blocking the pathways by which it acts and include atropine, cocaine, and ganglion blocking drugs.

Some drugs specifically antagonize the actions of 5-HT. They include reserpine, lysergic acid diethylamide (LSD), methysergide, phenoxybenzamine, morphine, cyproheptadine and are dealt with elsewhere in this book.

PLASMA KININS

The kinins are a group of polypeptides which have a potent action on smooth muscle and can be isolated from the tissues and the blood. They are formed from kininogen, a plasma protein, which is split by proteolytic enzymes to give bradykinin, a non-apeptide. These proteolytic enzymes include trypsin, various snake venoms and kallikreins which are enzymes found especially in the pancreas, saliva, blood and urine.

The plasma kinins have a very powerful vasodilator action causing a marked fall in blood pressure. They also increase capillary permeability. They cause a slow direct stimulation of extravascular smooth muscle (hence the name bradykinin) which is not antagonized by antihistamines or atropine. Nerve endings are stimulated to cause pain and there may be a release of nora-drenaline from the adrenal medulla. The action of the plasma kinins is transient as they are rapidly destroyed by kininases. Their function is not known, but may be to mediate the response to injury and inflammation. Aspirin has some opposing action to that of the kinins and the kininogen–kallikrein system overlaps with the blood-clotting mechanism as the Hageman factor (Factor XII) is common to both.

PROSTAGLANDINS

The prostaglandins (PG) are a family of related substances derived from a 20-carbon monocarboxylic acid, prostanoic acid. They have a 5-carbon (cyclopentane) ring with two hydrocarbon chains and small but critical variations in the 5-carbon ring divide them into the A, B, C, E & F series. Alphabetical and numerical subscripts to these letters further divide each series.

Although the prostaglandins were originally extracted from seminal plasma, they occur in the vast majority of tissues but their specific *in vivo* activity is not known for certainty in spite of a be-wildering array of investigations, the majority of which probably do not relate to the normal functions of the prostaglandins. They may promote ejaculation and assist the passage of spermatozoa in the female genital tract by causing movement of smooth muscle.

They may also play a part in inducing labour in human pregnancy. They relax the bronchi and vascular smooth muscle but contract the gut. They have metabolic functions especially on lipids and may have some transmitter function at synapses. There is marked species variation in the actions of the prostaglandins as well as large differences between the individual compounds.

Recent work has shown a very convincing relationship between the potency of the acute anti-inflammatory activity of drugs like aspirin and indomethacin and their ability to block the synthesis of PGE_2 and PGF_2. Work with paracetamol which has no anti-inflammatory activity has shown that, unlike aspirin and indomethacin, it will not block peripheral prostaglandin production (e.g. as in the dog spleen) but will do so in the brain in parallel with its antipyretic activity. Both aspirin and indomethacin are antipyretic and also block the brain biosynthesis of prostaglandins. This suggests that the clinical activities of the aspirin like drugs is determined by a differential sensitivity of the prostaglandin mechanisms of the target tissues (see page 189).

The therapeutic possibilities of the prostaglandins are potentially enormous now that their synthesis has been economically achieved. The major use so far has been in the induction of labour or abortion and various routes of administration have been tried from rectal, intravaginal, oral to intravenous.

Slow-reacting substance

Slow-reacting substance (SRS-A) appears in the perfusate of the guinea-pig lung after anaphylactic reactions. It produces a slow contraction of bronchial muscle and may play a part in human asthma. It is not antagonized by antihistamines.

ANGIOTENSIN

Changes in blood volume or sodium are monitored by the juxtaglomerular apparatus on the afferent arteriole close to its entry into the glomerulus. Low perfusion of the juxtaglomerular apparatus causes secretion of renin which acts on a circulating alpha-2 globulin angiotensinogen to split off the decapeptide angiotensin I which is rapidly converted by enzymes mainly in the lung to the active octapeptide, angiotensin II.

Angiotensin has many actions, the importance of which are controversial and some are probably extrarenal. It has marked pressor action due to vasoconstriction, but its role in hypertension is equivocal as the blood level of renin is not always related to the degree of hypertension. Angiotensin also enhances sympathetic nerve stimulation; stimulates ganglia, and releases catecholamines from the adrenal medulla.

The renin–angiotensin mechanism plays an important part in the control of the secretion of aldosterone (page 106) as angiotensin acts on the zonal glomerulosa of the adrenal cortex to cause secretion of aldosterone. Angiotensin also acts on the kidneys to lessen the renal blood flow so the glomerular filtration falls (an anti-diuretic effect) but it also inhibits tubular reabsorption of sodium (a diuretic effect).

Angiotensin has been used therapeutically as a pressor agent.

Disodium cromoglycate

This drug inhibits the degranulation of sensitized mast cells after challenge with antigen (Type I reaginic antigen/antibody reaction) and so prevents the subsequent release of histamine, 5-hydroxytryptamine and SRS-A.

Cromoglycate inhibits the release of these bronchoconstrictor substances only if present before the antigen challenge occurs and acts by stabilization of the membrane of the mast cell. It is of value in the prophylaxis of extrinsic allergic asthma and allergic rhinitis (i.e. due to extrinsic allergens such as pollens or house dust mites) but is not effective once exposure to the allergen has occurred.

Cromoglycate has no sympathomimetic, antihistaminic or corticosteroid effect and toxicity appears to be low. The drug is taken by inhalation or insufflation of the dry powder using a special dispenser, the spinhaler. Only a very small percentage of the drug administered is absorbed (around 5%) and this is rapidly eliminated unchanged in the urine and the bile, the effect lasting some 4–6 hours.

ERGOT ALKALOIDS

The ergot alkaloids are derivatives of lysergic acid found in extracts of ergot (*Claviceps purpurea*), a fungus growing on rye.

The various alkaloids have been purified and are of two main kinds: the amino acid alkaloids (peptides) such as ergotamine; and the amino alkaloids such as ergometrine. The main properties of vasoconstriction, oxytocic action and α-adrenergic block differ in the two groups and are summarized in Table IV.

Ergotamine

This is insoluble in water but soluble in alcohol. It has a moderate stimulant (oxytocic) action on the uterus but this is slow in onset. It has alpha adrenergic blocking actions, increased in the hydrogenated derivatives such as dihydroergotamine. The vasoconstriction produced by ergotamine makes it an effective drug in the treatment of migraine which is thought to be due to cerebral vasodilatation. Ergotamine may be given by most routes, though its side effects of nausea and vomiting may make it unusable in some people. The peripheral vasoconstriction has been known to cause gangrene and angina pectoris. The action of a single dose may be prolonged and cumulation rapidly occurs.

TABLE IV. The ergot alkaloids

Class of Compound	Vasocon-striction	Oxytocic Effect	α-Adrenergic Block
Amino acid alkaloids (peptides) Ergotamine Ergotoxine	+++	++ but delayed	+++
Amine alkaloids Ergometrine	±	++++, rapid, effective by mouth	Inactive

Ergotoxine

This drug is a mixture of three alkaloids, ergocristine, ergokryptine and ergocornine. Whilst of historical interest, it is not therapeutically important. Bromocriptine, a synthetic derivative of ergokryptine, is a dopaminergic-receptor stimulant and will inhibit prolactin release by the pituitary.

Ergometrine (ergonovine)

Ergometrine is a derivative of lysergic acid and aminopropanol and is water soluble. It is stable and active orally and its major action is oxytocic (i.e. stimulation of uterine muscle). The gravid uterus is especially sensitive at term or in the immediate post-partum period, when administration will cause long persistent powerful contractions. The actual type of contraction depends on the dose; moderate doses cause a faster contraction superimposed on a tonic contraction whereas higher doses cause a tonic contraction. In contrast, moderate doses of oxytocin produce slow generalized contractions with complete relaxation in between and high doses cause a tonic contraction. The sensitivity to ergometrine is low or absent in the first 6 months of pregnancy. On intravenous injection, ergometrine has its oxytocic effect in $\frac{1}{2}$–1 minute; in 2–4 minutes by intramuscular injection and in 4–8 minutes by mouth. The relative speeds of onset of action by these different routes may be of crucial importance in its therapeutic uses, which are: to prevent uterine haemorrhage; to aid delivery of the placenta, and involution of the uterus.

Ergometrine has few other effects on plain muscle and there is little vasoconstriction and no α-adrenergic blocking actions. It stimulates the central sympathetic system; is a 5-HT antagonist; and may give temporary but prolonged hypertension.

It is used mainly as the maleate (ergometrine maleate or methyl ergometrine maleate).

SPASMOLYTIC DRUGS

These drugs reduce the frequency and force of contraction of smooth muscle which, if excessive, can cause extreme pain. A spasmolytic drug may act at several sites and produce interference with the motor innervation at the ganglion or the nerve-effector junction or have a direct relaxant effect on the muscle fibre. Most of the spasmolytic drugs have been dealt with elsewhere in this book and a summary only will be given here.

1. Atropine-like drugs

These compete with the natural transmitter, acetylcholine, and occupy the receptors but do not trigger the muscarine-like actions. Atropine is the type drug and is dealt with on page 50. The atropine-like drugs include the naturally occurring belladonna alkaloids such as atropine and hyoscine and the related synthetic derivatives such as homatropine. There are many other synthetic atropine-like drugs, none of which has marked overall advantages when compared with atropine. They are less effective against vagal effects than against injected cholinergic drugs perhaps due to a similar extrinsic and intrinsic mechanism as with histamine (page 88).

Quaternary compounds such as atropine methonitrate and hyoscine methylbromide produce similar peripheral effects to the parent compound but have less action on the central nervous system as they do not penetrate to the brain so easily. There are also some synthetic quaternary ammonium compounds such as propantheline and dicyclomine, which have antimuscarine-like actions.

There are marked differences in the sensitivity of the various muscarine-like receptors to atropine-like drugs and those of the salivary, bronchial and sweat secretion; the heart and the eye are the most sensitive. The typical side effects of dry mouth and blurred vision are therefore almost unavoidable if an action on the gut or bladder is wanted.

2. Adrenergic drugs

At some sites, adrenergic stimulation causes relaxation of smooth muscle. These sites include the bronchiolar muscle, the alimentary and urogenital tract and the eye. Systemic administration may cause tachycardia (though see salbutamol, page 66) and they are often used topically.

Bronchospasm. The relief of spasm of bronchial muscle is often of extreme urgency in conditions such as asthma. Relief can also be produced by reducing the swelling of the bronchial mucosa or loosening the sticky secretions within the bronchi. Various drugs are available such as adrenaline, isoprenaline, orciprenaline, ephedrine, methoxyphenamine, salbutamol, disodium cromoglycate, and aminophylline. The routes of administration vary from oral and by injection to the inhalation of metered doses of aqueous aerosol or powder.

Hydrocortisone and other corticosteroids are of life-saving

value in status asthmaticus especially if this is unresponsive to other drugs.

3. Drugs acting directly on smooth muscle

These include the xanthine derivatives (page 222); papaverine (page 148); and the nitrites (page 147).

4. The ganglion blocking drugs

These are discussed on page 53.

REFERENCES

Cannon, P. J. (1968) Antihistamines, *Practitioner*, **200**, 53.

Cuthbert, M. F. (ed.) (1973) *The Prostaglandins: Pharmacological and Therapeutic Advances.* London: William Heinemann Medical.

Quilliam, J. P. (1968) Spasmolytic drugs. *Practitioner*, **200**, 65.

Robson, J. M. & Stacey, R. S. (eds.) (1968) *Recent Advances in Pharmacology*, 4th edn. pp. 185–212, 213–246. London: Churchill.

The word hormone (Gk. *hormao*, impel) was introduced by Starling in 1905 to denote substances liberated by glands of internal secretion which are carried by the blood stream to other parts of the body to produce specific effects on tissues.

Hormones are unique when compared with other drugs in that they occur naturally in the body and have a function which may be upset by hypersecretion or hyposecretion. They and their synthetic analogues are used in replacement therapy in deficiency states; to exploit the advantages of overactivity; or their normal action may be blocked by suppression or the use of antagonists.

The precise mode of action of hormones is unknown for the major part and probably varies with the different hormones. Some hormones (e.g. insulin) facilitate transport of substrates into the target cell. Other hormones (e.g. adrenaline, corticotrophin, vasopressin, glucagon) stimulate the formation of cyclic AMP in the target tissue. Recently it has been suggested that some hormones act directly on genes and regulate protein synthesis at the nuclear level.

PITUITARY GLAND

The pituitary gland or hypophysis cerebri may be considered as two major hormone-producing parts, the anterior lobe (adenohypophysis) and the posterior lobe (neurohypophysis).

The Anterior Lobe

The anterior lobe or adenohypophyis produces a number of hormones, most of which produce their effects by acting on other endocrine glands. They appear to be released by releasing factors which are low weight polypeptides formed in the hypothalamus that travel to the anterior pituitary by the hypophyseal-portal system. The control of secretion is by a feed back system in which falling levels of circulating adenohypophyseal and other hormones provoke the secretion of the appropriate releasing factor.

1. Thyrotrophin (thyroid stimulating hormone, TSH)

This glycoprotein acts on the thyroid to cause cellular hyper-plasia, increased uptake of iodine and secretion of thyroxine. The amount released is controlled by circulating thyroxine levels acting on the hypothalamic release of Thyrotrophin Releasing Factor (TRF). Thyrotrophin may be used clinically to assess the power of the thyroid gland to respond to pituitary stimulation. The production of thyroid hormone is discussed on page 125.

2. Long Acting Thyroid Stimulator (LATS)

This hormone is distinct from TSH being slower in onset of action.

3. Growth Hormone (somatotrophin, GH)

This hormone acts on all tissues to promote their growth. Administration causes an acceleration of bone growth but not bone age, unlike the sex hormones which cause both an accelera-tion of bone growth and an increase in bone age with premature fusion of the epiphyses. Administration of growth hormone also causes an increase in protein synthesis and a fall in the blood non-protein nitrogen and urinary excretion of nitrogen. There is a rise in the blood glucose and the glucose tolerance falls. There is also a loss of body fat.

Underproduction of growth hormone before puberty results in pituitary dwarfism. Over production is usually associated with an eosinophil adenoma of the pituitary and causes giantism if the epiphyses have not united and acromegaly after they have united.

Growth hormone is extremely species specific and the therapeutic uses are limited. As it is a protein, it must be given parenterally.

4. Gonadotrophins

Effective secretion of gonadotrophins does not begin till puberty (which they initiate). They also control and regulate the development of the gonads and secondary sex characters.

(i) *Follicle stimulating hormone (FSH)*. This glycoprotein stimulates the formation of the ovarian follicle in the female and spermatogenesis in the male.

(ii) *Luteinizing or Interstitial cell stimulating hormone (LH, ICSH*. In the female, this hormone is concerned with the maturation of the ovarian follicle, ovulation and the formation of the corpus luteum. In the male, it stimulates the interstitial cells of the testes to secrete androgens.

(iii) *Prolactin (lactogenic hormone; luteotrophin)*. This hormone helps to maintain the secretory effect of the corpus luteum in some animals but probably not in man. It initiates the production of milk after parturition, though other hormones such as the adrenal corticosteroids, growth hormone and thyroid hormone are probably necessary for the maintenance of lactation.

Non-pituitary gonadotrophins. Some gonadotrophins are secreted by tissues other than the pituitary. Chorionic gonadotrophin, which is mainly luteinizing, is secreted by the placenta and is found in the urine shortly after the start of pregnancy. It is the basis of such pregnancy diagnostic tests as the Ascheim–Zondek, Friedman and Xenopus. It is also secreted by various tumours such as hydatidiform mole, chorionepithelioma and testicular teratoma.

Pregnant Mare Serum Gonadotrophin (PMS) is found in the serum of pregnant mares and is of endometrial origin. It has both follicle stimulating and luteinizing action.

The gonadotrophins must be given by injection and have been found of use in the treatment of cryptorchism, infertility, and delayed puberty.

5. Corticotrophin (adrenocorticotrophic hormone, ACTH)

Corticotrophin is a polypeptide containing 39 amino acids and has a molecular weight of 20 000. Its function is to stimulate the release and synthesis of the adrenocorticosteroids, especially hydrocortisone (cortisol). It has less effect on the secretion of sex hormones and very little effect on the production of aldosterone (see page 106). The control of the secretion of corticotrophin is by the hypothalamic feed back system involving Corticotrophin Releasing Factor. If the blood level of adrenal corticosteroid is high, the secretion of corticotrophin is depressed and vice versa. Corticotrophin Releasing Factor (CRF) may also be released by any nervous stimulation, trauma, endotoxin, stress or anxiety. In the normal person there appears to be a diurnal variation in corticosteroid release with high levels in the early morning and low levels in the late evening due to a similar variation in ACTH release. The variation in ACTH secretion is probably secondary to variations in CRF production.

Uses of corticotrophin

(i) *Diagnostic*: corticotrophin may be given to test the function of the adrenal cortex and its ability to respond to stimulation by measuring the rise in urinary 17-hydroxy corticoids or 17-keto-steroids.

Corticotrophin produces a fall in the ascorbic acid content of the adrenal cortex, which provides a sensitive bioassay method in animals.

(ii) *Therapeutic*: corticotrophin is given to obtain adreno-cortical effects or to stimulate an inactive adrenal cortex. It does not cause muscle wasting as it stimulates both the secretion of androgens (which are anabolic) and hydrocortisone (which is catabolic). Hydrocortisone, given on its own, can cause muscle wasting as the catabolic action is now predominant.

Individual corticosteroids, however, can give more or less selective responses (page 109) and may be given in high doses, in contrast to corticotrophin which cannot give a selective response and can raise the blood level of adrenal hormones only to the maximum secretion capacity of the adrenal cortex (about four times the resting value). Corticotrophin is not active by mouth and, as it is a peptide, may cause sensitivity reactions.

Tetracosactrin. This is a synthetic polypeptide very similar in structure to corticotrophin. It stimulates the adrenal cortex and may also be used to assess adrenocortical function. It is less likely to cause allergic reaction than the natural product.

The Posterior Lobe

The posterior lobe or neurohypophysis produces two hormones, oxytocin and vasopressin. These are formed in the neurones of the supraoptic and paraventricular nuclei of the hypothalamus and are bound to a carrier protein, neurophysin. This neurosecretory material passes along the axons to terminate near the capillaries in the infundibular process. The hormones are released by increases in the osmotic pressure of the blood and perhaps by volume changes. They are also released by various physical and mental stresses such as haemorrhage, suckling and coitus. The afferent pathway is to the cell bodies and not the neurosecretory terminals and there is evidence of differential secretion.

1. *Oxytocin.* This hormone is an octapeptide and is available as a synthetic preparation. It is biologically standardized using the isolated uterus of the rat in dioestrus. Oxytocin is very similar chemically to vasopressin, but the synthetic preparation shows very little antidiuretic action and no pressor activity.

Oxytocin causes a rapid increase in the tone and motility of the uterus especially in the presence of oestrogens probably by an effect on electrical and contractile activity. Small doses initiate uterine contractions and increase their frequency but high doses cause a maintained increase in tone. The sensitivity of the uterus is maximal at term and may play a part in the normal process of labour.

The reflex secretion of oxytocin by suckling also causes liberation of milk by contraction of the breast myo-epithelium and oxytocin may be of use in the treatment of post-partum breast engorgement.

Oxytocin is rapidly absorbed and quickly excreted, the kidneys and liver playing a major role in metabolism. Pregnant women may also have an inactivating aminopeptidase in their plasma. Apart from its uterine and mammary effects, oxytocin may also cause coronary vasodilatation and a fall in blood pressure. If given in large doses over a period, its antidiuretic action may cause enough water to be retained to cause water intoxication.

The major use of oxytocin is to induce labour for which it is given by slow intravenous infusion. It cannot be given by mouth as it is destroyed, but can be given intramuscularly, subcutaneously or sublingually, though control by these routes is not likely to be so effective as by intravenous methods.

2. *Vasopressin (antidiuretic hormone, ADH)*. This is also an octapeptide differing in only two amino acids when compared with oxytocin. There is some species difference and arginine-vasopressin is obtained from man and cattle, and lysine-vasopressin (lypressin) from pig and hippopotamus.

The major action of vasopressin is to reduce the free water clearance by the kidney. In the absence of vasopressin, the distal convoluted tubules and collecting ducts are virtually impermeable to water but become freely permeable when vasopressin is present. Vasopressin may also constrict the vasa recta which will reduce the medullary blood flow and so increase the solute gradient. The release of the hormone is controlled by osmoreceptors in the hypothalamus, which are sensitive to changes in the solute osmotic pressure of the blood, and, if this rises, vasopressin is released and water retained. Release of the hormone is also caused by nicotine (and smoking), haemorrhage, and emotional disturbances. If the osmotic pressure of the blood falls as after the ingestion of water, less hormone is secreted and diuresis occurs. Release is also directly inhibited by alcohol which together with the drinking of large amounts of fluid explains the diuresis of the drinker.

Vasopressin also constricts smooth muscle and causes a rise in blood pressure, bronchoconstriction, intestinal colic and stimulation of the bladder, though larger doses are necessary than to produce a diuretic effect. It is of no value as a pressor agent as it also causes coronary vasoconstriction. Vasopressin contracts the non-pregnant uterus especially if this be previously sensitized by the giving of oestrogens.

Clinically, vasopressin is used mainly to control the urine output in diabetes insipidus in which there is insufficient production of the natural hormone. Because no reabsorption then occurs in the collecting tubules, the daily urine output may be as much as 10–20 litres. Vasopressin is inactive by mouth and is given parenterally or as a snuff. Lypressin may be used as a nasal spray.

ADRENAL CORTEX

The adrenal cortex secretes a large number of hormones which are steroid in structure. The steroids form a large group of compounds found both in plants and animals. They include oestrogens, androgens, progesterone, the adrenocortical hormones, the bile acids, cholesterol, vitamin D and its precursors. They are based on the ring structure given in table V which shows the structure of hydrocortisone. The adrenal steroids have a large number of actions which it is difficult to relate to a single physiological process. The available evidence suggests that the induction of protein synthesis is the major but not necessarily the sole pathway of their action. It is thought that the steroid enters the target cell and combines with a cytoplasmic aporeceptor which is able to recognize subtle differences in steroid structure thus conferring selectivity on the binding process. The steroid–receptor complex enters the cell nucleus and enhances mRNA and rRNA transcription with subsequent synthesis of specific proteins which ultimately mediate the physiological effects of the hormone.

The hormones of the adrenal cortex are divided for convenience into three groups: those having important effects on intermediary metabolism (glucocorticoids), those having principally salt-retaining activity (mineralocorticoids), and the sex hormones. The distinction between these groups is somewhat artificial and each has, to a varying extent, the actions of every group.

They are synthesized ultimately from cholesterol under the influence of corticotrophin and are degraded in the adrenal gland, the sex glands and the liver. Excretion is mainly in the urine as conjugates with glucuronic acid or as sulphates. The glucocorticoids form the 17-hydroxycorticoids, and the sex hormones the 17-ketosteroids, and these may be estimated in the urine.

The Mineralocorticoids

These hormones control the homeostasis of body electrolytes. They increase renal absorption of sodium and chloride and decrease their loss in sweat and gastrointestinal secretions. They increase the renal excretion of potassium by increasing its exchange for sodium in the tubules. The mineralocorticoids therefore cause retention of sodium and chloride with loss of potassium.

There are three mechanisms controlling mineralocorticoid secretion. The renin–angiotensin mechanism (page 94) and another negative feedback loop involving plasma potassium concentration are probably of equal importance. Corticotrophin is also concerned but to a lesser degree (page 103).

1. Aldosterone

This is the most important mineralocorticoid with only slight glucocorticoid action. The concentration can increase greatly in some causes of ascites and oedema due to cirrhosis of the liver and in some causes of cardiac oedema.

Spironolactone (page 176). This is a synthetic steroid which can block the action of aldosterone and is of use in cases of oedema associated with aldosterone excess. Aldosterone synthesis may also be inhibited by various drugs, such as aminoglutethimide (page 112).

2. Corticosterone

This is a natural steroid with moderately powerful mineralocorticoid actions. It also has glucocorticoid actions.

3. Desoxycorticosterone (deoxycortone)

This is a naturally occurring steroid, but synthesized and marketed as the acetate (DOCA). It is given sublingually as it is destroyed on passage through the liver.

The Glucocorticoids

The glucocorticoids are secreted by the adrenal cortex under the influence of corticotrophin (page 102), and circulate in the blood 95% bound to plasma protein. This binding may be to a globulin, corticosteroid-binding globulin (CBG) which has a high affinity but a low capacity, which means that though there is little of it, the hormones are tightly bound although reversibly. The concentration of CBG may rise when oestrogen levels rise as in oral contraception or during pregnancy. The concentration of CBG falls in liver cirrhosis, the nephrotic syndrome and in multiple myelomatosis. The glucocorticoids are not all bound to CBG with equal affinity and this is inversely proportional to their activity. Hydrocortisone has a high affinity and is much less active than dexamethasone whose affinity is low.

Albumen also binds corticosteroids and has a high capacity but a low affinity.

The actions of the glucocorticoids

1. *Protection in stress.* Glucocorticoids protect the body in conditions of stress, i.e. any physical injury, infection, or psychological strain which upsets the balance of body function. The mechanism of this protection is not known but is probably at the cellular level.

2. *Effect on reactive processes.* The glucocorticoids inhibit or suppress most inflammatory responses of a toxic, allergic or infective origin though this relief is symptomatic only and not curative of the original disease. They have a very important immunosuppressive action (page 299) associated with the ability to cause involution of lymphoid tissue. They have a lymphopenic action, but little effect on antibody formation in man, though this may be considerably depressed in the rabbit.

3. *Effect on carbohydrate metabolism.* They have a diabetogenic action by antagonizing insulin and inhibiting the uptake of glucose by the peripheral tissues. Gluconeogenesis is stimulated due to increased protein catabolism in the liver. Liver glycogen is increased in contrast to diabetes mellitus in which it is decreased.

4. *Effect on protein metabolism.* Protein synthesis is depressed, catabolism increased and a negative nitrogen balance may result with muscle wasting and increase in urinary uric acid axcretion.

5. *Effect on fat metabolism.* There is a mobilizing action on fat with a stimulation of free fatty acid (FFA) release. There is deposition of fat in the liver, shoulders, face and abdomen.

6. *Action on the kidney.* There is a variable mineralocorticoid action as well as a direct action on the nephron to enable it to respond to a water load by diuresis.

7. *Histomorphological action.* The glucocorticoids have a marked action on tissues derived from primitive mesenchyme. They have little effect on cartilage, though they may inhibit the growth of epiphyseal connective tissue. They cause osteoporosis by reducing the effect of vitamin D, reducing the absorption of calcium and increasing its excretion. They inhibit the growth of

elastic tissue and skin. They also reduce the number of circulating eosinophils.

8. *Various effects*. The glucocorticoids have many other effects including an increase of gastric secretion, delay or wound healing and production of upsets of mental function.

The natural glucocorticoids

1. *Hydrocortisone (cortisol, Compound E)*. This is the principal glucocorticoid secreted by the human adrenal gland. It is available in many forms for parenteral and local application.

2. *Cortisone*. This has to be converted to hydrocortisone in the liver before it becomes active.

Synthetic modifications of the corticosteroids

Many synthetic modifications of the corticosteroids have been made to try to separate the mineralocorticoid and glucocorticoid actions with the ultimate intention of separating individual effects. This has not been achieved, but the relative properties in some synthetic derivatives have been markedly altered. Table V shows the relative potencies of some natural and synthetic corticosteroids, but the figures given are meant to be a guide only.

1. *Mineralocorticoids*. The natural hormone, aldosterone, is rarely given as such save in primary hypoadrenalism in which production is known to be deficient. The usual mineralocorticoid given therapeutically is the synthetic analogue fludrocortisone which, as the acetate, is active orally and needs to be given daily. Another synthetic analogue, deoxycortone pivalate, may be given intramuscularly and is absorbed slowly over a period of 2–3 weeks.

2. *Glucocorticoids*. Prednisone and prednisolone are synthetic analogues of cortisone and hydrocortisone respectively, in which the sodium-retaining power is diminished but the other properties enhanced. Methylprednisolone has an extra methyl group at carbon 6 and, in effect, is devoid of sodium-retaining power. Dexamethasone and betamethasone are about 25 times more potent than hydrocortisone in their anti-inflammatory action and also devoid of significant sodium-retaining action. Triamcinolone

TABLE V. Relative potencies of naturally occurring and synthetic corticosteroids.

hydrocortisone

Compound	Relative Anti-inflammatory Action	Relative Sodium Retaining Action	Structure Compared Hydrocortisone
Cortisone*	0·8	0·8	11 = 0
Hydrocortisone*	1	1	See above
Prednisone	4	0·8	1 = 2, 11 = 0
Prednisolone	4	0·8	1 = 2
Methylprednisolone	5	0	6-CH$_3$ in prednisolone
Triamcinolone	5	0	9 $\propto$ F, 16-OH in prednisolone
Dexamethasone	25	0	9 $\propto$ F, 16 $\propto$ CH$_3$ in prednisolone
Betamethasone	25	0	9 $\propto$ F, 16 β CH$_3$ in prednisolone
Aldosterone*	0	3000	18-aldehyde and no 17-OH
Corticosterone*	0·3	15	No 18, 19, (CH$_3$)$_2$ or 17-OH
Deoxycortone*	0	100	No 11 = OH or 17-OH
Fludrocortisone	10	100	9 $\propto$ F

* Naturally occurring corticosteroids.

also has marked anti-inflammatory power, but is more likely than the others to cause muscle wasting and weakness.

Therapeutic uses of the corticosteroids

They may be used as replacement therapy or as supplement therapy. Replacement therapy is used to compensate for insufficient endogenous secretion as occurs after adrenalectomy and in Addison's Disease. In supplement therapy, large doses are given to enhance certain of the normal physiological actions of the corticosteroids.

The glucocorticoids are used to treat inflammatory and allergic reactions; as immunosuppressive drugs, and they may be of life-saving value in many acute conditions of stress. They are palliative only and do not cure any condition save where it is due to lack of hormone.

Side effects. Unfortunately, high therapeutic dosage means increases in the other and unwanted actions of the corticosteroids, which after prolonged administration may cause a iatrogenic Cushing's syndrome. These side effects may be forecast and explained by referral to the normal actions.

Excessive mineralocorticoid actions cause oedema and hypertension due to retention of sodium and water.

Excessive glucocorticoid actions produce a typical picture of a patient who has gained weight from oedema and fat deposition especially on the back (buffalo hump) and pelvis. There is a characteristic moon facies due to deposition of fat and alteration of the skin with increased fragility of blood vessels. The muscles waste especially of the pelvis and thigh, and there may be osteoporosis, collapse of vertebrae and degenerative arthritis.

There may be impairment of carbohydrate metabolism in 5–10% of patients, of whom 25% develop frank diabetes mellitus. Most of those who get impaired glucose tolerance have a familial disposition.

The anti-inflammatory and anti-immune actions can cause latent infections (e.g. tuberculosis) to flare up with minimal symptoms.

The skin thins, becomes striated and there will be delays in wound healing. Peptic ulcer can develop perhaps due to the inhibition of the protective gastric mucus. Various mental changes can occur from euphoria to frank psychosis. There may also be abnormalities of the sex hormonal control causing hirsutes, amenorrhoea, and other interferences with gonadal function.

The administration of exogenous corticosteroids leads to a suppression of the endogenous secretion of the adrenal cortex and marked atrophy of the zona fasciculata due to interference with the feed-back mechanism (page 103) to the hypothalamic–pituitary axis. Substantial dysfunction can occur after only a few days' therapy and may persist for months or years after a course of adrenal corticosteroids especially if this was prolonged. Even though the adrenal cortex itself is back to normal size, it will not be stimulated in response to the usual stimuli to the pituitary mechanisms. Steroid therapy must be gradually tailed off and never stopped abruptly. Exogenous steroids may be necessary during any period of stress (e.g. surgical operation) for several years after a prolonged course of steroid therapy though it is probably desirable to check the responsiveness of the adrenal cortex by the use of corticotrophin or tetracosactrin.

Inhibition of the synthesis of the adrenal corticosteroids

Some compounds interfere with the synthesis of the steroid hormones and may have a place in the treatment of overproduction.

1. *Dicophane* (*DDT*). This substance, normally known for its insecticidal properties, also interferes with the synthesis of adrenal steroids.

2. *Metyrapone*. This drug inhibits 11-hydroxylation and causes a fall in the synthesis of hydrocortisone and a compensatory rise in the secretion of corticotrophin. This in turn leads to increased production of hydrocortisone precursors such as the 11-deoxy compounds which can be detected in the urine as 17-hydroxy-corticoids. Metyrapone may be used as a test of anterior pituitary function, but this presupposes the ability of the adrenal cortex to respond.

3. *o.p.' DDD*. The 11-deoxy compounds are biologically active but *o.p.' DDD* interferes with synthesis at an earlier stage and there is no accumulation of biologically active compounds. It is, however, very cytotoxic which limits its use to adrenal carcinoma.

4. *Aminoglutethimide*. This substance is an analogue of glute-

thimide and inhibits the conversion of cholesterol to 20α hydroxy cholesterol and so interferes with the synthesis of the corticosteroids at a very early state. It has been used for the treatment of Cushing's Syndrome and secondary aldosteronism. It is likely to cause skin eruptions and drowsiness.

SEX HORMONES

The natural sex hormones are steroid and found in the ovarian follicle, corpus luteum and placenta in the female, and in the interstitial cells of the testes in the male. Some sex hormones are formed in the adrenal cortex of both male and female. The male hormones are androgens, and the female hormones are the oestrogens and the progestogens.

Androgens

Testosterone is the natural androgen secreted by the interstitial cells of the testes under the influence of the Luteinizing Hormone (Interstitial Cell Stimulating Hormone). It is metabolized chiefly in the liver to androsterone which is weakly androgenic, and to etiocholanone which is inactive. These metabolites are found in the urine as part of the 17-ketosteroids.

Testosterone is responsible for the pubertal growth, development and maintenance of the male sex organs, secondary sex characteristics and for normal spermatogenesis. It will increase protein anabolism and bone growth, but causes closure of the epiphyses.

Androgens are also secreted by the adrenal cortex of both sexes, and from the ovaries in the female. They are not identical with the testicular androgens and are less potent.

Administration of androgens

Testosterone cannot be given orally as, although well absorbed, it is rapidly destroyed by the liver. Even injection of testosterone gives only transient effects, though when implanted as pellets the actions may be more prolonged.

Some testosterone esters have a longer duration of action and are suitable for injection or oral administration. Testosterone propionate, for example, has an action lasting 2–4 days.

Testosterone oenanthate, phenylpropionate, isocaproate and decanoate have actions lasting several weeks.

Other synthetic substitutes include methyltestosterone which is active by mouth though better given sublingually, and fluoxymesterone which is active by mouth and about five times as potent as methyltestosterone.

The most important use of androgens is in replacement therapy when normal secretion is low or absent. Androgens are also very effective as anabolic agents but this is limited in women by the virilization they produce (and of the fetus in pregnancy) even though attempts to separate the anabolic actions have been partially successful.

The anabolic effect may be useful in senile osteoporosis, general wasting diseases, in acute renal failure to delay uraemia from protein catabolism, in aplastic anaemia and in some breast cancers. The use of androgens in hypogonadal dwarfism runs the risk of premature epiphyseal closure though this effect may be used to advantage in treating active excessive growth.

The choice of anabolic androgens is large and typical ones are norethandrolone, nandrolone, methandienone and stanozolol.

Oestrogens

Oestradiol and the much less active derivatives oestrone and oestriol are the naturally occurring oestrogens. They are secreted by the ovary, placenta, adrenal cortex and testes. They are metabolized mainly in the liver to be excreted in the urine as glucuronides and sulphates.

The oestrogens are feminizing and are responsible for the normal development and maintenance of the female genital tract and secondary sex characteristics. They are also responsible for some pubertal growth and closure of epiphyses though are less potent in this respect than the androgens. The oestrogens are responsible for the maintenance of the proliferative phase of the endometrium during the menstrual cycle and together with progesterone, the secretory phase.

Administration of oestrogens

Oestradiol is inactive by mouth though may be given by injection. There is a vast number of synthetic oestrogens, which may be steroidal, such as ethinyloestradiol or non-steroidal such as stilboestrol. Both may be given by mouth but ethinyloestradiol is some twenty-five times more potent. Stilboestrol is cheap and effective though is likely to produce nausea, vomiting, headache and abdominal discomfort.

Other synthetic oestrogens are dienoestrol, hexoestrol, methallenoestril, chlorotrianisene and mestranol.

Oestrogens have many uses. They may be used to correct deficiency states, especially that occurring at the menopause where there is a lack of oestrogen secretion characterized by hot flushes and psychological upsets.

Oestrogens may be used in conjunction with progesterone to induce normal menstrual cycles in some types of amenorrhoea. They may also be used to inhibit lactation and in high doses will temporarily limit the growth of some hormone dependent carcinomas of the breast and prostate. Their use in oral contraception is discussed below.

Clomiphene citrate. This is a synthetic non-steroidal drug. It is readily absorbed by mouth and largely metabolized in the liver and excreted via the bile into the gut.

It has a weak oestrogenic action but also has some potent anti-oestrogenic properties. It induces ovulation in anovulatory women and regulates irregular ovulation, but is only effective if the hypothalamic-pituitary system is intact and the ovaries capable of responding to FSH.

It is used in the treatment of infertility in women caused by disorders of ovulation. It can cause overstimulation of the ovary to cause multiple ovulation and multiple pregnancy.

Progestogens

Progesterone is the naturally occurring progestogen and is secreted by the corpus luteum and by the placenta if pregnancy develops. Progesterone is metabolized in the liver to pregnanediol and excreted in the urine as a conjugate. It is responsible for preparing the uterus for implantation of the ovum by changing the proliferative phase to the secretory phase. It also prevents ovulation, reduces the activity of the uterine muscle and stimulates the development of the alveolar tissue of the breast.

Administration of progestogens

Progesterone is inactive by mouth but may be given intra-muscularly or as an implant. There are synthetic substitutes such as ethisterone and norethisterone which are active orally.

Apart from their use in oral contraception, progestogens have a variety of uses and are used mainly in habitual abortion and various functional menstrual disorders.

Oral Contraception

At present this term is effectively restricted to oestrogens and progestogens taken by the woman to prevent conception. Many compounds interfere with spermatogenesis but are not of use clinically as male contraceptives because of their toxic effects and potential genetic damage to the sperm.

In pregnancy, the high circulating levels of oestrogens and pro-gestogens act on the adenohypophysis to inhibit the release of gonadotrophins and so prevent ovulation thus barring further conception.

This of course does not affect the gamete itself but prevents its release (c.f. spermatogenesis inhibitors). It is possible to do this artificially but the best method of giving the hormones is of some dispute; there are several recommended regimens and many types of oestrogens and progestogens used which have varied actions not only to inhibit ovulation but also may prevent the passage of the spermatozoa or implantation. The principal oestrogens used are ethinyloestradiol or its 3-methyl ether, mestranol. The prin-cipal progestogens used are derivatives of 19-nortestosterone (e.g. lynoestrenol, norethynodrel, norethisterone, ethynodiol, norges-trel) or of 17 α-hydroxyprogesterone (e.g. medroxyprogesterone acetate, megestrol acetate).

1. *Combined.* Here both oestrogen and progestogen are taken from the 5th to the 25th day after the start of menstruation. Withdrawal bleeding will then occur in 1–4 days and the regimen resumed after an interval 5–7 days. Various regimens exist and special packaging techniques can minimize errors due to forgetful-ness as the woman takes numbered tablets every day but some of these at the appropriate time will be dummy tablets.

In some formulations of combined tablets, the progestogen is high but in others the proportion is more balanced.

2. *Sequential.* Here oestrogen is taken from the fifth day of the cycle for 14–16 days followed by oestrogen and progestogen for 5–7 days.

3. *Continuous low dose progestogen.* This method uses a constant low dose of progestogen which makes the cervical mucus toxic and impenetrable to spermatozoa. It has a high failure rate but is less likely to cause venous thrombosis and carbohydrate intolerance.

4. *'Morning after' regimen.* In this method high doses of oestrogens are taken for 4–6 days after intercourse to prevent implantation of a fertilized ovum either by damaging the blastocyst or by hastening its passage through the Fallopian tubes.

Pharmacology of the oral contraceptives

The precise effects of the oral contraceptives are not fully understood and depend on the particular method. The secretion of gonadotrophin-releasing factors by the hypothalamus and the release by the pituitary of both Luteinizing and Follicle Stimulating Hormone is decreased and so ovulation stops. The long-term effect of pituitary suppression is not known and normal ovulation usually occurs within a month or two of cessation of therapy though evidence is accumulating that prolonged pituitary inhibition is not uncommon even after relatively short courses of the oral contraceptives.

There appears to be little effect on the ovary itself and though the initial changes in the endometrium depend on the type of therapy, it eventually becomes thin, hypoplastic and unsuitable for implantation. Progesterone causes the cervical mucus to become thick, tough and impenetrable by spermatozoa.

Liver metabolism may become impaired, glucose tolerance may decrease and the control of diabetes mellitus upset. There is increased hormone binding by the plasma and the total plasma hydrocortisone and protein-bound iodine increase (though this latter is not necessarily associated with hyperthyroidism). Mood changes may occur such as tiredness and depression, as well as headache, nausea, vomiting, flushing, and weight gain due to fluid retention. An increase in libido is often found due to removal of fear of pregnancy but contrarily sometimes a decrease is found.

There is evidence that the use of oral contraceptives predisposes to deep vein thrombosis, pulmonary and cerebro-vascular thrombo-embolic phenomena especially if the oestrogen-dominated type is used. The risks of oral contraceptives in general, however, are probably less than those of pregnancy itself and the choice of a particular regimen is made dependent upon the circumstances of the woman and the adverse effects encountered and it may be necessary to change regimens till the most suitable one is found.

PANCREAS

There are two internal secretions of the pancreas: glucagon from the α-cells of the islets of Langerhans and insulin from the β-cells, and they both play an active part in the maintenance of the blood glucose level. After hydrolysis of carbohydrates in the gut, glucose (dextrose) is absorbed via the portal blood. Some of the absorbed glucose is changed in the liver and skeletal muscle to glycogen, some is changed to fat in the liver, and with the rest of the blood glucose forms part of a very complex metabolic cycle shown in Fig. 11. The normal blood glucose is 70–180 mg/100 ml and is dependent on a number of interacting factors. The sensors of the homeostatic control of the blood glucose level are largely unknown though the pancreatic β-cells and some hypothalamic cells are sensitive to the amount of glucose in the blood. The effectors include a large number of compounds both hormonal and non-hormonal.

1. *Glucagon.* This hormone, a polypeptide of 29 amino acid residues, is secreted by the α-2 cells of the islets of Langerhans although similar substances are produced by endocrine cells in the gut. It has a major function of ensuring, in conjunction with insulin, a constant level of glucose, free fatty acids and ketones in the blood. Glucagon increases the formation of glucose from liver glycogen via formation of cyclic AMP and activation of hepatic phosphorylase. It has no effect on muscle glycogen or tissue utilization of glucose but accelerates lipolysis, protein catabolism and gluconeogenesis.

The control of glucagon release may be due to the substrate concentration in the blood perfusing the pancreas but catecholamine release from the sympathetic nerves of the pancreas may also be involved. Glucagon can also stimulate insulin secretion though this insulinotrophic effect is inhibited by adrenergic activity or intracellular substrate deficiency.

Glucagon also has a powerful inotropic action on the myocardium not prevented by β-adrenergic blockade (page 72) though this action is not useful in the treatment of the chronically failing heart.

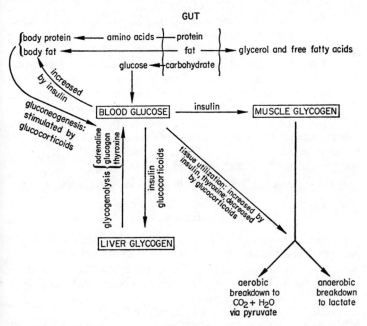

Fig. 11.

2. *Adrenaline*. Adrenaline increases liver glycogenolysis and so elevates the blood glucose level. Muscle glycogenolysis is increased and generates glucose-6-phosphate which elevates blood lactic acid. Adrenaline also raises the level of circulating free fatty acids. It does not antagonize the peripheral actions of insulin but does block insulin release.

3. *The adrenal steroids* (see page 105). The adrenal steroids, especially the glucocorticoids, are diabetogenic. They stimulate gluconeogenesis to form glucose from protein and amino acids; they increase liver glycogen but not that of muscle; they

antagonize insulin and inhibit the uptake of glucose by peripheral tissues and increase lipolysis from fat depots.

4. *Growth hormone* (see page 101). This hormone antagonizes insulin, so acromegalics are prone to diabetes and may even be insulin resistant. In hypopituitarism, conversely, there may be extreme sensitivity to insulin. Growth hormone may also play a permissive role in the action of glucagon.

5. *Thyroid hormone* (see page 125). This increases the requirement for insulin by increased gluconeogenesis, proteolysis and glycogenolysis.

6. *Diazoxide*. This compound is a thiadiazine analogue but, unlike chlorothiazide, is not a diuretic (page 173) and possesses marked hypotensive activity (page 152). Diazoxide also raises the blood glucose, mainly by a direct action on the pancreatic β cells to suppress the secretion of insulin but also perhaps by increased catecholamine release and increase of liver output of glucose. This hyperglycaemic action is quickly reversible unlike that of alloxan and may be used to treat severe idiopathic hypoglycaemia.

7. *Insulin*. Insulin is discussed in detail below.

Insulin

Insulin is a polypeptide hormone released by the β-cells of the pancreas. The factors controlling its release are not clear but the glucose concentration of the blood perfusing the pancreas is involved as well as glucagon, ketone bodies and possibly a duodenal factor, pancreozymin.

Insulin has a molecular weight of 5700 and consists of two polypeptide chains of 30 and 21 amino acids linked by two disulphide bridges provided by cystine. There is no species difference in the metabolic actions of insulin but there is some slight species variation in the amino acid composition; that of the pig resembling human insulin most closely. These differences can give rise to antigen–antibody reactions.

Insulin is destroyed by insulinase especially in the liver, kidney and pancreas and its biological half life is relatively short, only some 40 minutes. There is the equivalent of some 200 units of insulin in the pancreas but as a pancreatectomized man can live on 30–40 units a day, some of the endogenous natural insulin must be bound.

Insulin has a number of actions on metabolism which were thought to be by stimulation of carbohydrate metabolism but are now thought to be due to an increase in the permeability of the cell to glucose perhaps by removal of a transport inhibitor. This increased permeability increases tissue uptake and utilization of glucose but, even in the presence of insulin, the blood glucose level must be over a threshold of 70–90 mg/100 ml for uptake to occur. In the absence of insulin, whether by deficiency or antagonism, glucose will still be utilized, but the threshold for tissue uptake will be very high and glucose accumulates in the blood to give the characteristic hyperglycaemia of diabetes mellitus.

If this raised blood glucose level exceeds the renal threshold of about 180 mg/100 ml, glucose passes into the urine (glycosuria) and the consequent osmotic diuresis causes dehydration and electrolyte disturbances.

Insulin also increases the synthesis and storage of glycogen in peripheral tissues such as the heart and skeletal muscle though the intracellular concentration of glucose in the liver is dependent on the concentration in the perfusing plasma and is not directly altered by insulin. Insulin antagonizes gluconeogenesis, promotes tissue formation, stimulates amino acid incorporation and protein synthesis. Insulin also increases fat storage in adipose tissue by stimulating lipogenesis and inhibiting lipolysis so decreasing the plasma free fatty acids.

Diabetes mellitus (Gk. *dia*, through; *baino*, go)

The diabetic syndrome is due to a relative or absolute deficiency of insulin and is characterized by a rise in blood glucose. This hyperglycaemia causes glycosuria with a consequent osmotic diuresis and electrolyte and water depletion. There is also an increase in the mobilization of fat which is in part metabolized to give excessive amount of acetoacetic acid and derivatives in the blood (ketosis) and urine. The increase in gluconeogenesis causes a rise in urinary nitrogen and tissue wasting.

Although diabetes mellitus once meant these classical symptoms of polyuria, glycosuria, loss of weight and ketosis, there are minor degrees of carbohydrate intolerance and various stages of diabetes mellitus have been recognized.

Aetiology of diabetes. Numerous factors may be responsible for the diabetic state which is not always caused by a simple insulin deficiency and nearly all severe diabetics require more insulin than a pancreatectomized patient. Heredity, age, sex, obesity, infection and stress are all concerned. An insulin antagonist is any substance which interferes with the action of insulin and the anti-insulin actions of glucagon, adrenaline, adrenal steroids, growth hormone and thyroid hormone have already been discussed. Antibodies to endogenous insulin (auto-immunity) have been demonstrated in the serum of some patients.

A lack of production of insulin may be due to congenital absence or deficient reserve of pancreatic β-cells. Degeneration of β-cells may occur in carcinoma, haemochromatosis, pancreatitis or in the administration of alloxan. Some drugs may induce diabetes mellitus especially the thiadiazine diuretics though other diuretics seem not to do so.

Preparations of insulin

Insulin is used mainly to treat diabetes mellitus but may also be used to stimulate appetite; to produce hypoglycaemic convulsions in schizophrenics; and to treat hyperkalaemia (as insulin promotes the passage of glucose and potassium into the cell).

Although its structure is known, insulin is not commercially synthesized but is obtained from animals (mainly beef and pork insulins). It may be detected and assayed chemically though bioassay is often used such as by estimating the fall of blood sugar in rabbits or the production of hypoglycaemic coma in mice. Insulin has to be given parenterally as it is destroyed by gastric juice and there are a number of preparations available. These preparations are of two main types: those of short duration and relatively rapid action and those whose actions are slow in onset and last for long periods.

(a) *Insulin Injection B.P.* (*soluble insulin*). This is an aqueous solution of crystalline insulin and may be given subcutaneously, intramuscularly or intravenously. It has an onset of action within half an hour, maximal in 2–4 hours and lasting for 6–8 hours. It is obtainable as a solution containing 20, 40 or 80 units per ml. It is acid in reaction (pH 3·0) and there is a neutral preparation available (Neutral Insulin Injection) which allows slightly more rapid absorption and gives less discomfort on injection. The neutral preparation is available as either the beef or porcine form, which is useful if hypersensitivity develops to one form.

(b) *Insulin zinc suspensions.* These suspensions of insulin with zinc chloride are of several kinds differing in their time course of action and may be mixed in varying proportions and with Insulin Injection, if need be, to obtain a wide range of duration of effects. Known also as the lente insulins, they are available in two strengths containing 40 or 80 units per ml.

(i) Insulin Zinc Suspension (Amorphous) B.P. (Insulin Semi-lente). This has an onset of action in 1 hour which is maximal in 6–10 hours and lasts 12–16 hours.

(ii) Insulin Zinc Suspension B.P. (Insulin Lente). This is a mixture of the amorphous and crystalline forms and has an onset of action in 2–4 hours which is maximal in 8–12 hours and lasts 28–32 hours.

(iii) Insulin Zinc Suspension (Crystalline). B.P (Insulin Ultra-lente). This has an onset of action in 6–8 hours which is maximal in 16–24 hours and lasts for 36 hours.

(c) *Protamine Zinc Insulin B.P.* This is a suspension of insulin, zinc chloride and a suitable protamine. It has an onset of action in 3–6 hours, maximal in 14–20 hours and lasting for 24–48 hours. It may cause hypersensitivity reactions.

(d) *Isophane insulin, globin zinc insulin.* These preparations are little used and have a time course of action similar to that of Insulin Zinc Suspension.

Side effects of insulin therapy

These are mainly due to overaction with the development of hypoglycaemia. Hypersensitivity may occur and occasionally resistance may develop due to the formation of antagonizing antibodies.

Lipomata and fat atrophy can occur at the site of repeated injections and may cause erratic absorption.

Oral Hypoglycaemic Compounds

The diabetic syndrome (page 121) may be considered as due to relative or absolute deficiency of insulin action, and the pharmacological effects of an antidiabetic agent other than insulin should be considered in terms of its ability to increase insulin production and release by the pancreatic β-cells; to make insulin more effective; or to independently reproduce the metabolic actions of insulin. There are two main classes of drugs with an insulin-like action; the sulphonylureas and the biguanides.

1. The sulphonylureas

It has been known for some time that sulphonamides can cause hypoglycaemia and a similar group of compounds, the sulphonylureas, is used therapeutically for this purpose. They all have the general formula $R_1.SO_2.NH.CO.NH.R_2$ where R_1 is a benzene ring and R_1 is generally a simple three- or four-carbon chain. The chief differences between the various derivatives are in the speed of their absorption and elimination.

The sulphonylureas stimulate the pancreatic β-cells to produce greater amounts of insulin and inhibit the output of glucose from the liver. They are therefore of no use if the patient cannot make insulin and a history of ketosis is a contraindication to their use. The sulphonylureas may also stimulate the appetite, unlike the biguanides which are anorexic.

(i) *Tolbutamide*. This is readily absorbed and has a plasma half-life of 4–6 hours and needs to be given 2–3 times a day. It is rapidly converted by the liver to the inactive carboxytolbutamide and excreted via the urine and may give a false positive test for protein if the sulphosalicylic acid test is used.

(ii) *Chlorpropamide*. This drug is bound to plasma protein and has a much longer half-life (40 hours) than tolbutamide so needs to be given only once a day. It is little metabolized and is excreted via the kidney. Any metabolites also have hypoglycaemic action. It is more toxic than tolbutamide and there is a greater danger of hypoglycaemia. It may cause allergic rashes, jaundice, gastrointestinal upsets and an intolerance to alcohol similar to that of disulfiram.

(iii) *Acetohexamide; tolazamide*. These compounds are intermediate in duration of action and both have active metabolites.

(iv) *Glibenclamide*. This sulphonylurea has a prolonged action and needs to be given only once a day. It does not cause intolerance to alcohol like chlorpropamide.

2. The biguanides

There is general agreement that the biguanides do not lower the blood sugar in non-diabetic patients and that in the diabetic they will lower the blood sugar but do not cause clinical hypoglycaemia. They do not stimulate the release or production of endogenous insulin and may actually reduce it. They stimulate the peripheral utilization of glucose either directly or by facilitating insulin action. The presence of either exogenous or endogenous insulin is necessary for their continued efficient action. They may be used in combination with the sulphonylureas and the use of exogenous insulin avoided. The biguanides encourage weight loss though the reason for this is disputed. It may be due to loss of appetite but other mechanisms such as impaired glucose absorption, decreased fat synthesis have been cited. In normal doses biguanides do not appear to reduce the weight of obese non-diabetics.

(i) *Phenformin*. This drug is well absorbed from the gut and its actions last 6–15 hours. A sustained-release formulation is available which may give smoother control.

(ii) *Metformin*. This drug is little metabolized in the body and has a somewhat longer action than phenformin.

THYROID GLAND

The thyroid gland secrets three active hormones. Two of these, L-thyroxine (T_4) and L-tri-iodothyronine (T_3, liothyronine) stimulate metabolism, growth and development, raise oxygen usage and heat production. They are stored in the cavity of the follicles bound to a glycoprotein, thyroglobulin (colloid), and their production regulated by thyrotrophin (page 101).

The third hormone, calcitonin, lowers blood calcium and is formed in the C cells (parafollicular cells) which are not embryologically true thyroid tissue (page 130).

Mode of action

The thyroid hormones (i.e. thyroxine and tri-iodothyronine) have a complicated effect on growth, metabolic rate, water and ion transport, steroid and fat metabolism. It is unlikely that they act at a single metabolic control point and they could act at the nuclear DNA level to control the passage of information from DNA to messenger-RNA and so affect the rate of enzyme synthesis. If thyroxine is given, a rise in nuclear DNA is seen and subsequently a rise in protein synthesis. Increased enzyme synthesis increases the metabolic rate of cells and the time taken for this increased synthesis explains the delay of some days before the action of thyroid hormone becomes apparent.

Undersecretion of thyroid hormone causes cretinism in the young and myxoedema in the adult, characterized by a low metabolic rate, impairment of body processes and a failure of development in the child.

Oversecretion causes the clinical condition of thyrotoxicosis in which there is a raised metabolic rate with increase in heart rate, ventilation, oxygen usage and heat production. There may be associated protrusion of the eyeballs (exophthalmos), excessive nervousness and irritability.

Synthesis of thyroid hormone

Iodine is essential for the synthesis of thyroid hormones and is normally ingested in vegetables and fish. The need is for about 150 μg daily and it is present in the blood as inorganic iodide (less than 1 μg/100 ml) and as protein bound iodine or PBI (3–8 μg/100 ml).

Iodide is taken up preferentially by the thyroid in the iodide pump and is concentrated by energy requiring processes which are stimulated by thyrotrophin and inhibited by thiocyanate and perchlorate. In the next stage, inorganic iodide is oxidized by iodine peroxidase and added to tyrosine in several stages. Mono-iodotyrosine (MIT) and di-iodotyrosine (DIT) which are biologically inactive combine on the thyroglobulin molecule to form tri-iodothyronine (T_3) and thyroxine (T_4) which has four molecules of iodine. This conversion is blocked by the thioureas.

The thyroid hormones are released into the capillary lumen by autolysis of the thyroglobulin and attach themselves to an α globulin and to other proteins such as albumin and may be measured as Protein Bound Iodine (PBI). Tri-iodothyronine has less affinity for protein than thyroxine and so has a more rapid and shorter action. It has a half life of 2–3 days compared to the 6 days of thyroxine. The concentration of circulating hormone is in equilibrium with production and usage but may increase during pregnancy or oestrogen administration (e.g. oral contraception) as the Thyroxine Binding Globulin (TBG) increases. Blood thyroid hormone falls in conditions where there is a low plasma globulin and may be displaced by drugs such as the salicylates. The PBI is raised in thyrotoxicosis and lowered in myxoedema.

The Thyroid Gland in Therapeutics

The thyroid gland provides a lot of hormonal problems which basically may be thought of as deficiency of hormone or its overproduction.

1. Thyroid deficiency

This causes cretinism in the young and myxoedema in the adult and these two conditions are the only unequivocal indications for the use of thyroid hormone.

Thyroid extract is available (Thyroid Tablets B.P.) but its use is inadvisable as the potency of the tablets may vary. They are not only bioassayed by a non-standardized and unreliable technique but deteriorate on storage.

The two active thyroid hormones (thyroxine and tri-iodothyronine) have been isolated and are readily available. L-thyroxine sodium (Thyroxine Tablets B.P.) is probably the most useful but tri-iodothyronine (Liothyronine Tablets B.P.) is more potent and quicker in onset of action.

The initial dose of thyroid hormone should be small and be increased according to clinical progress. As the effects of a particular dose of thyroid hormone may take days to appear and several weeks to stabilize, changes of dosage should be at intervals of not less than a month or cumulative effects are likely and some months are often necessary before a stable euthyroid state is reached.

2. Thyroid overactivity

This is often associated with a goitre (which means simply an enlargement of the thyroid).

Simple goitre. Some goitres (simple, endemic, colloid) are not necessarily associated with signs of overproduction of hormone (thyrotoxicosis). The enlargement is due to some physiological interference with hormone production and the subsequent stimulation by thyrotrophic hormone to produce the normal amount of hormone. Many substances are known which interfere with the normal mechanism.

Absolute iodine deficiency may occur in areas remote from the sea and may be avoided by the addition of iodine to the ordinary table salt (1·5 mg iodine/100 g salt). Other causes are the ingestion of goitrogens in the food such as vegetables of the Brassica family (cabbage, brussels sprouts, turnips) or some drugs such as sulphonamides or PAS. Genetically determined deficiency of the enzymes required in thyroxine synthesis can also cause goitre.

Treatment with iodine may be all that is required, though thyroxine itself is often necessary. The goitre will regress with treatment, provided there has been no irreversible structural change.

Thyrotoxicosis. The treatment of thyrotoxicosis can be surgical and medical. Various antithyroid drugs are available to bring the patient to a euthyroid state when further treatment can be operative and a large part of the hyperactive gland removed. Maintenance therapy by antithyroid drug rather than operation is also used but must be continued for a year or so to minimize relapse, which is common.

(*a*) Iodine: paradoxically the administration of iodine to hyperthyroid patients produces a temporary remission of thyrotoxicosis and promotes involution of the gland, making it smaller, firmer and less vascular and so facilitating surgery. The symptoms of thyrotoxicosis recur within about a fortnight despite continuance of iodine, and this treatment is used mainly on patients for surgery perhaps after treatment with other antithyroid drugs. Iodine is usually given as tablets of potassium iodide though Lugol's Iodine (5% iodine and 10% potassium iodide in water) was much used.

(*b*) Radio-iodine (^{131}I, ^{132}I): the radioactive isotopes are treated by the body just like ordinary iodine and are similarly concentrated by the thyroid. They emit mainly beta rays with a small gamma component and destroy thyroid tissue. It is difficult to choose a dose which will destroy the required amount of tissue as different thyroid glands vary considerably in their sensitivity.

The effects of radio-iodine are slow and may take some months to reach a maximum. There is also a danger of destroying too much thyroid tissue and so producing hypothyroidism. The possible production of carcinoma and genetic damage also restricts the routine use of radio-iodine to patients over 45 years of age.

^{131}I has a half life of eight days so there is an appreciable radiation hazard and it is used mainly to treat hyperthyroidism and thyroid carcinoma. ^{132}I has a half life of 2–3 hours and is used (if essential) in children, pregnant women and also as a tracer to assess thyroid function.

(c) Potassium perchlorate: perchlorates (thiocyanates and nitrates) block the uptake of iodide by the thyroid. This blocking action can be overcome by excess iodide so perchlorates are of no use as antithyroid drugs before surgery if iodine is also to be used for the immediate preoperative treatment. Iodine may also be found in other drugs such as some cough mixtures.

Perchlorates are more liable than the other antithyroid drugs to cause aplastic anaemia and are usually used only in patients who are sensitive to the thiouracil compounds.

(d) Thiouracil compounds: It was noticed some 40 years ago that plants of the Brassica sp., such as cabbage and rape seed, could cause goitre due to the presence of thiourea.

Thiourea and the related thiouracil compounds cause considerable diminution of hormone synthesis by the thyroid which may not be obvious for some days due to the continued output of stored thyroxine. They do not block the uptake of iodide by the thyroid but prevent its incorporation in organic form by antagonizing oxidation by peroxidase and by blocking the coupling of iodotyrosines to form iodothyronines. There is considerable diminution in the amount of colloid in the thyroid follicles which become irregular and lined by highly cuboidal epithelium.

Thiouracil compounds do not cause any interference with the output of thyrotrophin by the pituitary which may even increase as the blood level of thyroid hormone falls.

These drugs are readily absorbed from the gut and widely distributed in the body and excreted via the urine. In pregnant women they will cross the placenta and may cause fetal goitre and, as they are also excreted via the milk, may also cause goitre of the suckling infant.

Other side effects include lymphadenopathy, arthritis, skin reactions and various blood dyscrasias especially agranulocytosis.

Thiourea and thiouracil, the original compounds, with methylthiouracil and propylthiouracil, have been superseded by carbimazole. They suppress the signs of thyrotoxicosis, and clinical improvement occurs in a week or so, though the patient may take several months to become euthyroid. The dose is then reduced to a level judged on clinical progress. If used alone, without subsequent surgery, relapse is common.

(e) Imidazoles. Like the thiouracil compounds, these drugs block the incorporation of iodine into amino acids. Carbimazole is the drug of first choice in thyroid overactivity but has a short duration of action (about 4 hours). Methimazole is also a member of this group. Toxic effects are rare, various skin rashes and nausea being the most common.

(f) Other drugs used in thyrotoxicosis: sedation or β-adrenergic blocking drugs may be useful to counteract the rise in heart rate and similar manifestations of thyrotoxicosis which, however, are probably due to a direct effect of excess thyroid hormone rather than sympathetic overactivity.

PARATHYROID GLANDS

In response to hypocalcaemia, these glands produce the parathyroid hormone which is a polypeptide of about 80 amino acids with some slight species variation. Its function is to keep the blood calcium constant by mobilizing calcium from bone, promoting its absorption from the gut and decreasing its excretion via the kidney, faeces, sweat and milk.

CALCITONIN

Calcitonin (thyrocalcitonin) is produced by the C cells (parafollicular cells) found in the thyroid tissue. These cells are not embryologically true thyroid tissue but derive from the ultimobranchial body.

Calcitonin is secreted in response to hypercalcaemia and lowers blood calcium by a direct effect on bone, inhibiting its breakdown. The importance of calcitonin is not at present fully assessed and it may play an important part in the regulation of the blood calcium level. It is a polypeptide and has been synthesized. It is available from human, porcine and salmon sources though there is marked species variation and activity in the structure. Calcitonin is of value in the treatment of Paget's disease of bone and some forms of hypercalcaemia.

REFERENCES

Foster, G. V. & McIntyre, I. (1968) Calcitonin. In *Recent Advances in Pharmacology*, 4th edn. Robson, J. M. & Stacey, R. S. (eds.) pp. 247–262. London: Churchill.

Catt, K. J. (1971) *An ABC of Endocrinology*, London: *The Lancet*.

11   The Vitamins

The vitamins catalyse metabolic processes and are often the main or sole component of a co-enzyme. They are supplied mainly in the diet though some (e.g. vitamin D) may be synthesized by the body. The vitamins are required in very small amounts and there is not always a clear distinction between them and other essential dietary constituents.

Deficiency of a vitamin causes symptoms which, though easy to recognize when severe, may be very equivocal in minor deficiencies. There is likely to be a need for several vitamins and essential minerals in deficient diets which can result in a very complex clinical picture. The role of subclinical vitamin deficiency in ill health is controversial, but the ingestion of large amounts of vitamins by persons on an otherwise adequate diet benefits no one but the manufacturer and chemist, and may be dangerous with vitamins A and D.

The young, the pregnant, and those with intestinal malabsorption may need supplements even with normal diets. The recommended dietary intake (see Table VI) varies with the authority and tends to reflect the purpose of the recommendation; whether to prevent signs of deficiency or to maintain optimum health. The recommended intake also varies according to the age and sex of the subject; the pregnant or lactating woman and young children will need proportionately more than the normal adult. Vitamins are commonly classified as the water soluble (such as the B group and ascorbic acid) and the fat soluble (such as vitamins A, D, K and E).

WATER-SOLUBLE VITAMINS

1. Ascorbic acid (vitamin C)

Ascorbic acid is a white water-soluble crystalline compound synthesized by most animals save man, monkey, and guinea-pig. It is a very active reducing agent and is easily and reversibly oxidized to dehydroascorbic acid. It is rapidly destroyed by heat, alkalis, copper, and plant oxidases. It is found especially in fresh fruit and green vegetables though is destroyed by cooking. Ascorbic acid is readily absorbed and is found especially in the liver, adrenals and pituitary though in trivial amounts. It functions in intracellular oxidation–reduction systems and in the formation of collagen.

TABLE VI. Daily requirements of the vitamins

Vitamin	Other names and equivalents	Approximate daily requirement (adult male)	Main dietary source
A		5000 IU	Fish, milk, egg yolk, liver
D	Calciferol (D_2) Cholecalciferol (D_3)	10–20 µg (4–800 units)	Fish, liver, egg yolk, butter, (sunlight)
Thiamine	B_1, aneurine	1–2 mg	Yeast, grain husks, peas, beans, eggs
Riboflavine	B_2	1–7 mg	Yeast, milk, meat, offal, vegetables
Pyridoxine	B_6	1–5 mg	Yeast, wheat germ, liver
Nicotinamide	Niacin, nicotinic acid	19 mg	Yeast, whole grain, meat, offal
Pantothenic acid		10 mg	Yeast, liver
Folic acid		50–100 µg	Yeast, liver, green vegetables
Cyanocobalamin	B_{12}	1–10 µg	Liver, kidney
Ascorbic acid	C	70 mg	Fresh fruit, green vegetables
K	Acetomenapthone, phytomenadione		Green leaves, fruit, Synthesized by intestinal bacteria

Deficiency of ascorbic acid causes scurvy which is characterized by swollen gums, cutaneous haemorrhages, general ill health, anaemia and delayed wound healing. Scurvy is rare in this country though is not unknown, especially in a subclinical degree in children, old people, and others with defective diets.

Ascorbic acid may be readily prescribed as tablets or as fresh fruit. Its usefulness as a cure for the common cold, when taken in massive amounts, is unproven.

2. The vitamin B group

These vitamins are commonly grouped under one heading due to the original historical distinction between the fat-soluble A vitamins and the water-soluble B vitamins.

(a) *Thiamine* (*vitamin B_1, aneurine*). This vitamin is found in the husks of grain such as rice and wheat; in peas, beans and eggs, and some may be synthesized by intestinal bacteria.

It acts as the co-enzyme for the decarboxylation of pyruvic acid and α keto-glutaric acid. Deficiency of thiamine causes the clinical condition of beri-beri characterized by polyneuritis, cardiac failure and mental disorder. Deficiency has also been implicated in some kinds of neuritis such as alcoholic neuritis and thiamine is often prescribed for these on perhaps scanty evidence.

(b) *Riboflavine* (*vitamin B_2*). This vitamin, an orange pigment composed of iso-alloxazine and ribose, is found in yeast, meat offals, milk, and green vegetables. It acts as the co-enzyme ribo-flavine adenine dinucleotide (FAD), a hydrogen carrier in various metabolic processes such as those involving the pyridine nucleotides and cytochrome systems.

Deficiency causes angular stomatitis, seborrheic dermatitis, and vascularization of the cornea.

(c) *Pyridoxine* (*vitamin B_6*). This is a pyridine derivative found in yeast, wheat germ, liver, muscle, vegetables and may also be synthesized in the large intestine. It is found in three intercon-vertible forms; pyridoxal, pyridoxamine and pyridoxine. It acts as a co-enzyme in many metabolic conversions of amino acids and may play a part in fat metabolism. It is not certain what pyridoxine deficiency produces in man, but, in rats, it causes red, swollen, and oedematous extremities.

(d) *Nicotinamide*. This is the amide of nicotinic acid and is found in meat, offal and grain. Nicotinic acid acts as a co-enzyme either as diphosphopyridine nucleotide (NAD) or triphosphopyridine nucleotide (NADP) and serves a vital function in tissue respiration.

Severe deficiency produces pellagra with the three classical signs of diarrhoea, dermatitis, and dementia. Both nicotinamide and nicotinic acid may be used to treat deficiency but nicotinic acid has a direct action on blood vessels to cause vasodilatation and itching of the skin.

(e) *Pantothenic acid.* Pantothenic acid is converted to coenzyme A in the body. It is not clear what are the results of deficiency in man but there are characteristic lesions in lower animals.

(f) *Cyanocobalamin and folic acid.* These vitamins are essential for the maturation of the red cell (page 157).

FAT-SOLUBLE VITAMINS

1. Vitamin A

Vitamin A is a long-chain alcohol found in fish, milk, egg yolk and liver. It is also found in carrots and the green leaves of vegetables as a precursor or provitamin, β-carotene, which structurally is two molecules of vitamin A joined together.

Vitamin A is concerned in the formation of the retinal pigment, visual purple or rhodopsin, which is a protein complex containing vitamin A. In deficiency of the vitamin there will be reduction of vision in poor light (night blindness) as the pigment will not be synthesized in adequate amounts. Deficiency also causes morphological changes of various epithelial surfaces. The sebaceous glands and hair follicles become blocked with keratin (follicular keratitis); the tear glands of the eye cease to function, and there may be heaping up of the epithelium on the scleral conjunctiva (xerophthalmia). If the cornea becomes affected (keratomalacia), blindness may result.

Vitamin A may be given as cod-liver oil, halibut oil, and foods such as margarine are often fortified with it.

2. Vitamin D

Vitamin D includes several substances derived from steroids, either naturally or artificially. The natural vitamin (D_3) is formed from 7-dehydrocholesterol and is found in fish liver oils and (to a much smaller extent) in egg yolk and butter. Man is able to synthesize it in the skin by the action of sunlight on 7-dehydrocholesterol and this is a major source of the vitamin.

If ergosterol is artificially irradiated, vitamin D_2 (calciferol) is formed and is usually indistinguishable in effect from the natural vitamin. Ingested vitamin D requires the presence of bile for its absorption; it is stable and not destroyed by normal cooking.

Vitamin D has several important functions. It promotes absorption of calcium from the gut as well as having a direct effect on the growth of bone and cartilage.

Deficiency causes the clinical condition of rickets or its counterpart in adults, osteomalacia. The bones are deficient in calcium and phosphorus and become soft and liable to bend with failure of normal epiphyseal development and ossification. Blood calcium may fall low enough to cause tetany and there may be a compensatory overactivity of the parathyroid which worsens the rickets by mobilizing calcium from the bones to maintain the blood calcium level. Overdosage of vitamin D is harmful and may easily occur if the correct preparation and dosage for the particular type of deficiency is not used. The consequent hypercalcaemia can cause ectopic calcification, nephrocalcinosis and renal failure.

3. Vitamin K

This vitamin is essential in the production of certain factors concerned with the clotting of blood. It is discussed on page 162.

REFERENCE

Marks, J. (1968) *The Vitamins in Health and Disease.* London: Churchill.

DIGITALIS

The word digitalis is both a specific and generic term and may be used to include all drugs with a digitalis-like action as well as extracts from the foxglove. Digitalis-like compounds are found scattered throughout animal and plant life and include the poisons found in the skin and parotid glands of some toads, the Monarch butterfly, Lily of the Valley and squill. Ouabain is obtained from the seeds of *Strophanthus gratus*.

The classical digitalis is obtained mainly from the foxglove (*Digitalis purpurea*) and is a crude mixture of the active substances (called cardiac glycosides) and various inert substances such as saponins. Although standardized extracts are available such as Digitalis Tablets B.P., it is now more common to use the purified cardiac glycosides like digoxin (from *D. lanata*) and digitoxin (from *D. purpurea*). These cardiac glycosides may be broken down into a sugar and an aglycone or genin (see diagram below).

The aglycone has a sterol skeleton (cyclopentaperhydrophenanthrene ring) with an unsaturated lactone group at carbon-17 which may be 5 membered (a cardenolide) or 6 membered (a bufadienolide). The aglycones have a digitalis-like activity but are much less potent than the parent glycoside.

The sugar is usually a monosaccharide attached at carbon-3 and may be responsible for the power of fixation to cardiac tissue and the water solubility of the cardiac glycosides.

The centres classically associated with digitalis-like action are an OH (or sugar) at carbon-3, an OH at carbon-14 and the unsaturated lactone group at carbon-17. Recent work may much modify this simple viewpoint. All digitalis compounds are very similar in structure with only minor modifications of the molecule, but they may be very different in the time course of their actions. Digoxin, for example, differs from digitoxin solely by having an OH at carbon-12 but the half life of digoxin is 1·8 days compared to the 9 days of digitoxin.

The basic structure of the cardiac glycosides.

Absorption and metabolism of digitalis

Taken orally digoxin is 80% absorbed, digitoxin is wholly absorbed and ouabain is absorbed little if at all. Contrary to previous belief, digitalis is not selectively localized in the heart but very rapidly disappears from the blood on intravenous injection and is found mainly in the liver, spleen and kidneys. Metabolism occurs mainly in the liver and, in man, significant amounts are excreted via the urine.

There is a whole range of time courses of action of the various digitalis compounds. The onset of action depends on the firm binding of the drug to the myocardium, and the time for this to occur differs greatly with different compounds. This latency of action occurs even with intravenous administration. The firmness of binding also varies and is inversely related to the elimination and hence the duration of action.

On intravenous injection digoxin, for example, will have an effect that is maximal in ¾–3 hours and gone in 1–2 days whereas digitoxin will not have its maximal effect for up to 8 hours and may still have noticeable effects for several weeks. At the other end of the scale, acetyl strophanthidin which is an aglycone, if given intravenously, exerts an affect which is maximal in 15 minutes and lasts only 4 hours.

The Actions of Digitalis

Digitalis has actions on the heart and other tissues and these are summarized:

1. Actions on the heart

(a) *Increase in contractility.* Digitalis has a positive inotropic action, that is, increases the contractility of the heart. Although open to some dispute, contractility may be defined as the capacity of a muscle to do work at a fixed length. It has been argued that digitalis acts only on the failing heart (see below) but recent evidence shows that it acts on normal hearts also.

(b) *Effect on conduction.* Digitalis has marked effects on conduction either directly on the conducting tissue or indirectly via the vagus.

Digitalis slows conduction through the atrioventricular node and bundle of His and increases their refractory period. This does not slow the normal heart as the recovery of the conducting tissue is still fast enough for all impulses to be propagated until atrioventricular block is produced. If, however, the a-v node is being excited at an abnormally fast rate (see atrial fibrillation, page 141), slowing will occur as some of the impulses reach the a–v node during the refractory period of the previous impulse.

The effect via the vagus (the indirect effect) is more marked at lower doses of digitalis and slows the heart. There seems to be a direct action on the vagal nucleus as well as a peripheral sensitization to the effect of vagal stimulation (i.e. acetylcholine) though other mechanisms have been proposed. This vagal action is blocked by atropine. With higher doses of digitalis the extravagal (direct) effect predominates and this is not abolished by atropine.

There is also an interaction between the sympathetic drive to the heart and digitalis though the exact mechanism is not clear.

(c) *Automaticity*. High doses of digitalis increase the automaticity of the heart's conducting system (i.e. the ability to develop spontaneous activity).

(d) *Excitability*. Digitalis increases the excitability of the heart, i.e. the ability to respond to a stimulus. High doses, however, may depress excitability.

2. Actions other than on the heart (extracardiac actions)

Digitalis increases the contractile force of skeletal muscle, venous and arterial smooth muscle. This vasoconstrictor action is especially marked in the hepatic veins of dogs.

Digitalis may also have a slight direct action on the renal tubules, decreasing reabsorption and so increasing the elimination of sodium and water.

The basic mode of action of digitalis

This is complex and incompletely known. Digitalis was thought to have little effect on myocardial oxygen consumption until toxic effects occurred. Recent work has shown, however, that any increase in myocardial contractility increases oxygen usage, but, when the heart is considered as a pump, the total oxygen consumption is also influenced by other factors such as intramyocardial tension, the velocity of shortening and the heart rate.

In congestive failure (see below), the dilatation of the heart greatly increases its resting oxygen consumption which falls when digitalis reverses the dilatation. This fall may so outweigh the rise caused by the increased contractility as to result in a net reduction of oxygen usage with a consequent rise in the mechanical efficiency of the heart.

The significance of digitalis on ion movements is not clear, and it is not possible to relate unequivocally the increase in myocardial contractility with any particular change. Digitalis appears to have a specific action on membrane ATPase and inhibits it in a similar range of concentrations required for an inotropic effect. The ATPase is concerned with active membrane transport of sodium and potassium and its inhibition causes a rise in the intracellular concentration of sodium and a fall in that of potassium. It seems doubtful that therapeutic concentrations of digitalis cause appreciable lowering of intracellular potassium though may do so in toxic doses. A low serum potassium level, as may be found when using some diuretics (page 176) makes toxic effects more likely.

Increased uptake of calcium is also concerned in the inotropic action of digitalis and the calcium ion is critical in excitation–contraction coupling. High serum calcium has a potentiating effect on the inotropic action of digitalis.

The actions of digitalis in the diseased heart

(a) *Congestive heart failure*. Starling's law shows that the heart will respond, within limits, with increased work when increased demands are made on it. If, due to disease, the heart cannot cope with the work demands of normal life, this results in congestive heart failure. This is characterized by dilatation and decreased force of contraction of the heart, reduced cardiac output, venous congestion and oedema.

Digitalis reverses these symptoms, decreasing venous pressure and the dilatation of the heart by increasing cardiac output. The renal blood flow increases and a vigorous diuresis occurs which decreases the blood volume and the oedema. The slowing of the failing heart after digitalis is due mainly to the improved cardiac function and consequent reduction in sympathetic drive rather than to the direct effects of digitalis.

(b) *Atrial fibrillation*. This is characterized by a chaotic disturbance of the atrial wall with asynchronous contraction of the various parts of the atria at about 500/minute. The ventricle cannot respond efficiently and its contractions are irregular in force and rhythm, and the function of the heart is grossly impaired.

Digitalis depresses atrioventricular conduction and so lessens the number of impulses passing to the ventricles which then contract more slowly and efficiently. Digitalis also so improves myocardial function that a reversion to sinus rhythm may occur.

The toxic effects of digitalis

Digitalis is a very potent drug but has a low therapeutic ratio and toxic effects are easily produced. Digitalization, which could be defined as the required clinical response, needs some 60% of the minimum toxic dose which is itself about 50–80% of the minimum lethal dose. The incidence of toxic effects is a reflection of the low therapeutic ratio and of the use of the minor toxic signs to show that digitalization is complete. The use of a fixed dosage schedule rather than titration against clinical response and of diuretics which produce hypokalaemia are important contributory factors.

In man, the toxic effects may be considered in two groups: the cardiac toxic effects and the others. They are not always easy to diagnose and much clinical acumen is needed.

The cardiac toxic effects are the most important by far and may cause almost any form of arrhythmia. The effect of digitalis on conduction, the increase in excitability and automaticity contribute to the block of the normal impulse path and the development of ectopic centres of excitation.

The frequency of the different types of arrhythmias is variable but ventricular premature beats, often as coupled beats, are the most common, followed by partial to complete atrioventricular block with more complex ventricular arrhythmias and ventricular fibrillation as the terminal event.

The electrocardiogram may be used to indicate the presence of digitalis but is not much use in a quantitative fashion, though T wave changes are very roughly proportional to dosage. The T wave becomes lower, diphasic and then negative (i.e. displaced in an opposite direction to the QRS) and the ST segment may become scaphoid. The PR interval will be prolonged. The changes caused by therapeutic doses of digitalis must be distinguished from the abnormalities caused by toxic doses.

The other toxic effects of digitalis include gastrointestinal disturbances such as anorexia, nausea, vomiting, diarrhoea and salivation, perhaps due as much to medullary stimulation as to an effect on the stomach. Various other toxic effects include neurological disturbances, skin rashes, muscle cramps and changes in colour vision. True allergy to digitalis is rare.

With regard to the administration of digitalis and the avoidance of toxic effects, it is still pertinent to quote William Withering, who wrote in 1785 '. . . let the medicine therefore be given in the doses and at the intervals mentioned above; let it be continued until it either acts on the kidneys, the stomach, the pulse or the bowels; let it be stopped upon the appearance of any of these effects and I will maintain that the patient will not suffer from its exhibition, nor the practitioner be disappointed in any reasonable expectation. . . .'

Treatment of digitalis toxicity. The first step in the treatment of digitalis toxicity is to stop the drug. Supplemental potassium may reverse some arrhythmias though may aggravate conduction defects. If other drugs are being used which cause depletion of intracellular potassium (such as the thiadiazine diuretics), they should be stopped. The potassium may be given by mouth or intravenously (as the chloride).

The lowering of serum calcium by the use of citrates or ethylene diamine tetra-acetic acid (EDTA) decreases myocardial irritability and favours the re-entry of potassium into the cells.

Recent work on β-adrenergic blocking drugs such as propranolol shows great promise in the treatment of digitalis toxicity and maintenance therapy with propranolol may increase digitalis tolerance. The mode of action of propranolol is complex and includes its β-adrenergic blocking action and its quinidine like properties. Other anti-arrhythmic drugs, e.g. phenytoin, bretylium (page 146) may also be of use.

Preparations of digitalis

The most commonly used preparations of digitalis in the United Kingdom are the cardiac glycosides digoxin and digitoxin, though some people still use extracts of digitalis leaf (Prepared Digitalis Tablets B.P.). Other countries may show different preferences.

The glycosides are pure but extracts of leaf need to be biologically standardized. The various methods used are based on the principle of comparing similar toxic effects and assuming that these are related to the therapeutic action in the same way. The official British Pharmacopoeia method (1973) is to infuse the unknown preparation into anaesthetized guinea pigs or pigeons until the heart is arrested and repeating this in other groups of the same species using a standard preparation of digitalis. By simple proportion the strength of the unknown solution may be calculated.

ANTI-ARRHYTHMIC DRUGS

The rhythm of the heart is very complex and depends on the regular, spontaneous generation of waves of excitation from a pacemaker which is normally situated in the sino-atrial node. Intracellular recordings show a slow diastolic depolarization in the pacemaker which, when it reaches a threshold, initiates an action potential. This action potential spreads to the atrioventricular node and down the bundle of His to the ventricular tissue to initiate contraction of the cardiac muscle.

Other nodal tissue also shows this 'diastolic drift' but, normally, this is slower than that of the sino-atrial node which consequently reaches the take-off potential first and so controls the heart rate. In some circumstances control may shift to other parts of the conducting system. This is in contrast to the steady diastolic membrane potential of ordinary cardiac fibres which may, however, develop diastolic drift if injured and be able to generate ectopic impulses.

Abnormal impulse generation causes irregular rate and contraction of heart. These arrhythmias are of many forms depending on the precise nature of the ectopic foci of excitation.

There are two major groups of drugs available to counteract arrhythmias. Some such as quinidine, procainamide, lignocaine and phenytoin act by a direct membrane stabilizing action to raise the threshold of the myocardium to excitation so that a greater diastolic drift is necessary for the initiation of action potentials and may also prolong the refractory period of the myocardium to lessen the possibility of premature re-excitation from adjoining areas. The other group of drugs is the adrenergic receptor or neurone blocking type such as propranolol or bretylium.

Quinidine

Quinidine is one of the cinchona alkaloids and the dextrorotatory isomer of quinine, to which it is very similar in its pharmacological actions (page 280).

It is toxic to unicellular organisms and is also an antimalarial, an antipyretic, an oxytocic, and a muscle depressant. By far its most important actions are those upon the heart where it is used to prevent and stop various arrhythmias.

Quinidine slows myocardial conduction and depresses myocardial excitability and the rate of initiation of pacemaker potentials especially those of ectopic sites. The effective refractory period of the conducting system (when the threshold to excitation is high) is greatly increased though the resting potential, the duration of the action potential and the absolute refractory period (during which no stimulus will excite) are not much affected.

Quinidine has a blocking action on the cardiac vagal system (a vagolytic action) similar to but less than that of atropine so that vagal stimulation will no longer slow the heart. Indeed, in man the heart rate may rise due to the vagal block. Quinidine depresses the contractility of the cardiac muscle and the arterial blood pressure may fall due to peripheral vasodilatation and depression of the vasomotor centre.

Quinidine has other actions which may be of therapeutic importance. It stimulates and then depresses the central nervous system; it has a curariform action on skeletal muscle, and by mouth will irritate the gut.

The mode of action of quinidine is not known but is probably by stabilizing the cell membrane by inactivating the carrier mechanism which transports sodium across the membranes during excitation.

Quinidine is well absorbed by mouth and is excreted in the urine both unchanged and as a breakdown product. It can also be given intramuscularly or intravenously but is likely to cause hypotension if given by the latter route.

Quinidine is used therapeutically to stop and prevent various arrhythmias such as atrial fibrillation, paroxysmal tachycardia, extrasystoles or, in conjunction with digitalis, to convert atrial flutter or fibrillation to normal rhythm.

Quinidine is a toxic drug and may cause hypersensitivity reactions. It may also cause tinnitus, deafness, nausea and vomiting (cinchonism). There is also considerable risk of producing ectopic beats, a–v block or even cardiac arrest.

Procainamide

Procaine itself is a local anaesthetic and has some quinidine-like actions. It is also rapidly destroyed and is convulsant (page 243).

A derivative of procaine, procainamide, is more stable and exerts an antiarrhythmic action in doses having little effect on the central nervous system. Procainamide is absorbed via the gut and can be given by injection. It is mainly excreted unchanged via the urine and, unlike procaine, is not broken down by plasma esterase.

The pharmacology of procainamide is very similar to that of quinidine but it has much less depressant action on myocardial contractility. It also has anticholinergic, ganglion blocking and local anaesthetic properties. Whilst its central nervous actions are not marked, large doses can cause tremors. Intravenous administration may provoke hypotension and collapse.

Lignocaine (page 243)

This local anaesthetic is particularly useful in the treatment of arrhythmias due to myocardial infarction or digitalis but is not effective in suppressing supraventricular arrhythmias.

Phenytoin

This anticonvulsant drug (page 203) is effective in abolishing digitalis-induced arrhythmias. When given intravenously, phenytoin may cause hypotension, heart block, cardiac or respiratory arrest.

Propranolol

This β-receptor blocking drug (page 72) has very marked anti-arrhythmic effects and is probably the drug of choice in those arrhythmias due to digitalis or sympathetic over-activity. Its anti-arrhythmic action is more likely to be due to its β-receptor blocking properties than its membrane stabilizing action. The L- and the D-isomer are equipotent with regard to membrane stabilization but only the L-isomer is effectively anti-arrhythmic which parallels its β-blocking properties.

Bretylium

This adrenergic neurone blocking drug was originally used in the treatment of hypertension but this use is now obsolete. It does have a useful anti-arrhythmic action especially to treat ventricular arrhythmias due to myocardial infarction or to digitalis overdosage.

VASODILATOR DRUGS

Only drugs acting directly on the vessel wall are discussed here. Drugs acting at sites like ganglia, the adrenergic receptor or neurone are dealt with elsewhere.

Nitrates and Nitrites

Aliphatic nitrites (such as amyl nitrite), inorganic nitrites (such as sodium nitrite), organic nitrates (such as glyceryl trinitrate), but not inorganic nitrates, relax smooth muscle to cause a generalized dilatation of arterioles, capillaries and venules. The blood pressure falls precipitously and the heart rate increases due to baroceptor reflexes. These drugs also relieve smooth muscle spasm in the urinary, biliary, alimentary and bronchial tracts.

1. *Amyl nitrite*. This drug was first used by Lauder Brunton in 1867 for the relief of angina pectoris. It is an inflammable, volatile and pungent liquid dispensed in cloth-covered glass capsules (vitrellae) which are broken and the vapour inhaled so that absorption takes place in the lungs. There is a marked vaso-dilatation especially of the blush area. Headache may be caused by dilatation of the meningeal vessels. The fall in blood pressure causes a strong reflex tachycardia and dizziness which is accentuated in the upright position. The response is abrupt and short lived.

2. *Glyceryl trinitrate* (*nitroglycerin*). This is an oily explosive liquid made up in non-explosive tablets which are allowed to dissolve under the tongue so that the drug enters the systemic circulation without delay or destruction in the liver. Its action is maximal in several minutes, lasting up to an hour, and is less abrupt and intense than that of amyl nitrite.

3. *Long-acting nitrates*. Drugs such as pentaerythritol tetranitrate are of disputed value, but this drug, for example, can be swallowed and is said to have a vasodilator action in 10 minutes which lasts for 5 hours.

Mode of action of the nitrites

This is obscure but there is some evidence that nitrate is first converted to nitrite. They may also have a direct metabolic and anti-adrenergic effect. The major use of the nitrites is in the treatment of angina pectoris which is discussed below.

Tolerance soon develops to the nitrates and the nitrites though this is rarely a problem as it is abolished by a few days of abstinence from the drug.

Papaverine

This drug is an isoquinoline derivative found in opium (page 181) but is not an analgesic. Unlike morphine, which causes spasm of smooth muscle, papaverine is a smooth muscle relaxant. Its action is not very powerful and does not last long so it is not of much use. Papaverine may be used if local vasodilatation is required as, for example, in peripheral arterial spasm when it is injected into and around the vessel.

Xanthine Derivatives

These are dealt with on page 222.

Angina Pectoris

Cardiac muscle is supplied with blood via the coronary arteries and the normal extraction of oxygen is almost complete. The only way for the myocardium to get more oxygen is to increase the coronary flow which is normally done by dilatation of the coronary arteries as anoxia is the most potent stimulus to dilatation.

Relative ischaemia and failure to deliver enough oxygen to the myocardium may be caused by spasm, thickening, complete or partial thrombosis of the coronary arteries as well as extra-coronary causes such as anaemia. This relative ischaemia can cause the typical pain called angina pectoris or, if severe enough, will lead to the death of the cardiac muscle supplied by that vessel (myocardial infarction). By dilating the coronary arteries with drugs such as glyceryl trinitrate, it has been postulated that the coronary flow will increase and the relative ischaemia relieved. Whilst this happens in the healthy experimental animal, it has been questioned if dilatation of pathologically thickened vessels is possible, besides which it is likely that tissue anoxia will already have maximally stimulated any responsive vessels. The cause of the undisputed relief of anginal pain by the nitrites is probably due to the pooling of blood in the capacitance vessels, decrease in venous return and fall in blood pressure with a consequent reduction in cardiac work and oxygen usage though the precise mode of action is disputed. Whether any anti-adrenergic or metabolic effects play a part is not known with certainty.

Other drugs used in angina include sedatives, β-adrenergic blocking drugs and anticoagulants. The β-adrenergic blocking drugs such as propranolol, practolol and oxprenolol (page 72) appear to act by blocking sympathetic impulses to the heart which slows. The blood pressure and the cardiac output fall and so cardiac work (and oxygen consumption) decreases. They also reduce the cardiac response to exercise.

The place of the anticoagulants in the long or short term treatment of coronary insufficiency is controversial and will not be discussed here.

HYPERTENSION

Hypertension or high blood pressure is difficult to discuss and details should be sought in the standard texts. The aetiology is usually uncertain and complex and there is no general agreement on the dividing line between a high blood pressure and normal values. It is agreed that high blood pressure is harmful and to lower it may be beneficial.

The body control of blood pressure is complex and includes the renin–angiotensin mechanism (page 94) and aldosterone–sodium chloride retention (page 106). Disorders of these mechanisms can result in hypertension and appropriate therapy be instituted. Rarely can the cause of the hypertension be treated save in such cases as unilateral renal disease, Conn's tumour and phaeochromocytoma. The treatment of hypertension is usually a symptomatic one based mainly on the lowering of the tone of various vascular beds by influencing their autonomic control. Fig. 12 shows the major sites of action of these antihypertensive drugs but, as most of them have been dealt with elsewhere in this book, it is proposed only to summarize their actions.

It is well perhaps to distinguish between drugs which will lower the blood pressure and those which are of use in hypertension. The nitrites, for example, produce a marked postural hypotension but the effect is transient, accompanied by a reflex compensatory tachycardia so is not of clinical use.

1. *Veratrum alkaloids*. Alkaloids from *Veratrum* sp. have a complex pharmacology. They act on excitable structures to lower the discharge threshold and so cause repetitive firing. The number

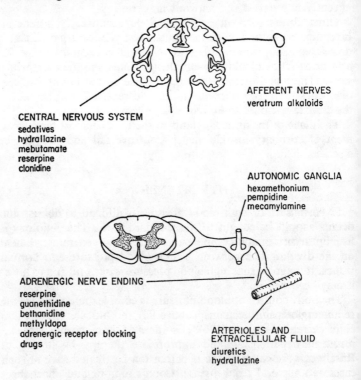

AFFERENT NERVES
veratrum alkaloids

CENTRAL NERVOUS SYSTEM
sedatives
hydrallazine
mebutamate
reserpine
clonidine

AUTONOMIC GANGLIA
hexamethonium
pempidine
mecamylamine

ADRENERGIC NERVE ENDING
reserpine
guanethidine
bethanidine
methyldopa
adrenergic receptor blocking
drugs

ARTERIOLES AND
EXTRACELLULAR FLUID
diuretics
hydrallazine

Fig. 12. Sites of action of antihypertensive drugs.

of vagal afferent impulses received by the brain from the baroceptors of the carotid body and carotid arch is increased and is interpreted as denoting a higher pressure than actually exists. The vagal tone is raised and the sympathetic tone lowered by the negative feed back mechanism that maintains blood pressure homeostasis and will cause a fall in blood pressure.

Unfortunately the nausea and vomiting caused by the veratrum alkaloids seems inseparable from the hypotensive effects and they have not been as useful as was hoped.

2. *Reserpine.* This drug has both central sedative and peripheral adrenergic neurone blocking action (pages 68, 228).

3. *Clonidine.* This imidazoline derivative (page 71) has been recently introduced for the treatment of hypertension and may also be used in migraine. The fall in blood pressure caused by clonidine is thought to be due to a reduced sympathetic outflow from the central nervous system perhaps by stimulation of central α- adrenergic receptors connected to inhibitory pathways. There is no evidence of an effect on brain amines. Intravenous clonidine may cause a transient rise of blood pressure due to peripheral α-receptor stimulation before the prolonged centrally caused fall.

As homeostatic reflexes are largely undisturbed, clonidine produces little postural hypotension, but may cause sedation and dry mouth.

4. *Hydrallazine.* This drug was thought to act centrally but it is more likely that the hypotensive action is due to peripheral vasodilatation. It is not very useful clinically due to severe toxic effects.

5. *Mebutamate.* This drug is thought to act by depressing brain stem vasomotor centres and spinal vasoconstrictor pathways. The antihypertensive action is weak and may be merely a placebo or sedative action. Mebutamate is closely related to meprobamate, a tranquillizer (page 229).

6. *Ganglion-blocking drugs.* These are dealt with on page 53. They are little used these days save in anaesthetic practice or in the emergency reduction of blood pressure.

7. *Adrenergic neurone-blocking drugs.* These drugs such as guanethidine, bethanidine and methyldopa (page 68) are, at the present time, the drugs of choice for the treatment of hypertension.

8. *Adrenergic receptor-blocking drugs.* α-blocking drugs such as phenoxybenzamine cause an unpredictable postural hypotension due to the abolition of peripheral vasoconstriction but, as the β-receptors are not affected, there may be a marked compensatory tachycardia. Sometimes patients may become resistant to adrenergic neurone-blocking drugs because of extreme sensitivity to circulating noradrenaline. If phenoxybenzamine is given as well, it may be possible to control the blood pressure.

β-blocking drugs such as propranolol have a hypotensive effect.

They will control the blood pressure in both the erect and the prone position with no marked upsets of the gut or sexual function.

9. *Diuretics.* Chlorothiazide and similar diuretics (page 173) have an antihypertensive action. This is not due solely to the diuresis and reduction of blood volume but may also be due to a direct action on the blood vessels.

Diazoxide is also a thiadiazine derivative but, unlike chlorothiazide, is not a diuretic and will cause water and sodium retention. It will also raise the blood glucose (page 120). Diazoxide has a potent hypotensive action which is not associated with pronounced postural hypotension and when given intravenously will cause a marked fall of blood pressure in 30 seconds which may last for 2–24 hours. The mode of action does not appear to be by interference with sympathetic activity but by a direct action on the precapillary resistance vessels rather than the postcapillary capacitance vessels. This direct hypotensive action is similar to that possessed by the thiadiazine diuretics but is much more marked.

Diazoxide may be used to lower the blood pressure in hypertensive crises but its prolonged use results in sodium retention and hyperglycaemia.

REFERENCES

Blinks, J. R. & Koch–Weser, J. (1963) Physical factors in the analysis of the actions of drugs on myocardial contractility. *Pharmacological Review*, **15**, 531.

Glynn, I. M. (1964) The action of cardiac glycosides on ion movements. *Pharmacological Reviews*, **16**, 381.

Parratt, J. R. (1969) Pharmacological aspects of the coronary circulation. In *Progress in Medicinal Chemistry*, **6**, 11. Ellis, G. P. & West, G. B. (eds.). London: Butterworth.

Trautwein, W. (1963) Generation and conduction of impulses in the heart. *Pharmacological Reviews*, **14**, 277.

13   The Blood

ANTI-ANAEMIA DRUGS

The word anaemia implies a reduction in the amount of circulating haemoglobin usually associated with a fall in the number of red cells. It is useful to have some form of classification when considering treatment.

Anaemia may be caused by excessive loss as in haemorrhage; or by excessive destruction as in the haemolytic anaemias. Anaemia may also be caused by a failure of the blood-forming sites to make blood due to destruction, depression or replacement of the bone marrow as occurs in carcinomatosis, exposure to X-rays or the administration of such drugs as chloramphenicol. Blood may also fail to form normally if there is a deficiency of the factors required for haemopoiesis. These factors include iron, vitamin B_{12}, folic acid, ascorbic acid and thyroxine. Some anaemias may be the result of several factors operating together and iron deficiency anaemia, for example, may be caused by chronic slight haemorrhage in which the loss of iron is greater than the ability of the body to absorb iron from the diet.

Iron

Iron is an essential factor for normal haemopoiesis and is found especially in liver, egg yolk, spinach and peas but not in fish, chicken, milk or white bread. The average diet supplies about 10–20 mg of elemental iron daily of which perhaps only 5–10% is available for absorption as the rest forms insoluble complexes with phytates and phosphates in the alkaline medium of the lower intestines. Approximately 20–40% of the iron in the food is released by the digestive processes especially in the duodenum and upper small bowel and then passes into the mucosal cell. Ferric iron (Fe^{+++}) is not so well absorbed as the ferrous form (Fe^{++}) but is reduced to ferrous by substances in the food such as ascorbic acid. Haem iron is taken up by the mucosal cell as the complex molecule but is then broken down by xanthine oxidase to release Fe^{++}.

The Fe^{++} in the mucosal cell may pass either rapidly across to the serosal pole and so to the blood or combine in the cell with apoferritin to form ferritin dependent on the iron status of the individual and the rate of erythropoiesis. It seems that the mucosal cells are coded during their formative stages in the Crypts of Lieberkuhn by the amount of iron entering them. Excessive iron entering the mucosal cell from the gut is not passed on to the blood but is kept as ferritin to be eventually passed out in the faeces when the cells are exfoliated after a life of 3–4 days. This control of iron absorption is by what has been called the 'ferritin curtain'.

Iron circulates in the plasma as a complex with the glycoprotein β_1 globulin 'transferrin' (siderophilin) which has two sites for iron transport. If both are filled (i.e. the iron stores of the individual are high) they are more reactive than if only one site is filled (i.e. iron stores low) and transferrin passes more easily back to the mucosal cell to stop further absorption. The transferrin system could bind more than 3 mg iron/litre of blood but normally has only 0·8–1·7 mg/litre and so is only partially saturated.

The total body iron is about 3–5 grammes, of which haemoglobin iron forms some 60–70% (i.e. 2–3 grammes) and the rest is in ferritin, cytochrome and myoglobin. There is some 930 grammes of haemoglobin in the body (15·5 grammes/100 ml of blood) of which 0·3% is elemental iron, i.e. 100 ml of blood contains about 50 mg of iron.

The average life of the red cells is about 120 days, so less than 1% is destroyed each day. This represents a release of about 20 mg of iron but most of this is re-used for haemopoiesis. The actual loss of iron by the human male is about 1 mg daily and occurs via the urine, skin and hair. The loss in the female is more uncertain and in the menstruating woman may be up to 2–3 mg daily as the menstrual flow forms a major source of loss. Whilst this flow is often about 50 ml (25 mg of iron), it could easily rise to 250 ml (125 mg of iron). The need for iron will also increase markedly in pregnancy and lactation as the foetus requires some 200–400 mg of iron, as well as the loss in the placenta, and during childbirth and lactation. There is some saving due to the amenorrhoea of pregnancy so the net loss may be negligible or as much as 500–700 mg. The average woman and growing child will therefore require about 15 mg of iron daily and the average man about 5 mg. This is supplied by a good diet, though in people with poor nutrition, the margin is narrow.

The administration of iron

Iron deficiency is characterized by a microcytic hypochromic anaemia. It may be caused by an inadequate intake especially in women of reproductive age, in inadequately weaned babies or poorly cared for elderly people. It may be found in malabsorption syndromes such as coeliac disease, steatorrhoea and after partial gastrectomy. Chronic loss of blood is especially likely to cause iron deficiency anaemia and the loss of 10 ml of blood daily (a mere two or three teaspoonfuls) can cause a greater loss of iron than can be made up from the diet. Iron may be administered orally or parenterally.

Oral administration of iron. The merits of various forms of oral iron are controversial but if allowance is made for personal bias and advertising, it is probable that ferrous sulphate is as good as any other compound if equal amounts of elemental iron are given, and it is certainly cheaper than most. It is essential when comparing iron compounds to do so by the actual amount of available iron and not by tablet size. The most commonly used forms of oral iron are:

(i) Ferrous Sulphate Tablets B.P. 200 mg (60 mg elemental iron).
(ii) Ferrous Gluconate Tablets B.P. 300 mg (36 mg elemental iron).
(iii) Ferrous Fumarate Tablets B.P. 200 mg (65 mg elemental iron).
(iv) Ferrous Succinate Tablets B.P. 100 mg (35 mg elemental iron).

There are other forms of iron available. These include slow-release compounds where ferrous sulphate is slowly liberated in the duodenum or upper jejunum: iron chelates such as ferrous aminoacetosulphate or sodium iron edetate; and mixtures such as Ferric Ammonium Citrate Mixture B.P.C. Many iron preparations are marketed with additives such as vitamins and trace elements but there is no convincing evidence of the superiority of these preparations over the simpler forms of iron, and indeed some of them are potentially dangerous, such as those containing folic acid.

The major toxic effects of oral iron are gastrointestinal upsets such as nausea, vomiting, diarrhoea and the production of black stools. Their occurrence seems essentially related to overdosage (more than 300 mg of iron daily) though some people are intolerant.

The haemoglobin should rise 1–2% daily during oral iron treatment, which should be carried on for a couple of months after the blood picture is back to normal to replenish the body stores which become very depleted even before the haemoglobin level starts to fall.

Parenteral administration of iron. This may be needed if there is a proven malabsorption (e.g. in coeliac disease); if the patient is incapable of being trusted to take oral iron; if there is a genuine intolerance to oral iron or late in pregnancy to replenish the stores. There is no evidence that the haemoglobin level rises faster than by the oral route.

(i) Intravenous preparations: these include saccharated iron oxide in sucrose and dextrin colloidal ferric hydroxide which contain 20 mg iron/ml. Though usually given at intervals over a period, some people advocate the total dose infusion technique in which the calculated necessary total amount of iron is given slowly over 5–6 hours. This may cause immediate reactions such as hypotension, dyspnoea and vomiting, so a preliminary test dose is advisable.

(ii) Intramuscular preparations: both Iron Dextran Injection B.P. and Iron Sorbitol Injection B.P. are suitable and contain 50 mg elemental iron/ml. The injections are painful and may stain the skin. Iron Dextran has been found to cause sarcoma in rats and mice though this does not yet seem to have occurred in man.

Iron poisoning. The side effects of iron therapy have been discussed above but it also is often the cause of poisoning in young children who mistake the attractive colours of the tablets for sweets. The ingestion of excessive amounts of iron causes gastric haemorrhage, circulatory collapse and death. It is treated by desferrioxamine mesylate which chelates iron to form a non-irritant complex and is given intravenously, intramuscularly, and intragastrically after lavage with 1 % sodium bicarbonate.

Megaloblastic Anaemias

Folic acid, cyanobalamin (vitamin B_{12}) and ascorbic acid are concerned in the metabolism of purines, pyrimidines and the eventual synthesis of nucleoproteins. If there is a deficiency of these substances, a macrocytic anaemia will result typified by large red cells in the blood stream. Some macrocytic anaemias (e.g. due to certain bone marrow disorders) are normoblastic and the cells are merely more primitive and hence larger and less mature than the normal red cell. In macrocytic anaemias due to deficiency of vitamin B_{12} or folic acid, the cells are megaloblastic, that is, there has been interference with the normal processes of erythropoiesis and abnormal cells are produced. The effects of the deficiency are not confined to the bone marrow and there are effects on gut epithelium, skin, hair and myelination of the central nervous system.

The cobalamins

These are porphyrin-like ring structures with an atom of cobalt at the centre, resembling in many details other natural molecules such as haem and chlorophyll. Cyanocobalamin (vitamin B_{12}) has a cyanide radical though cobalamins with other radicals such as hydroxocobalamin are effective in haemopoiesis. Cyanocobalamin was isolated in 1948 from the liver where it occurs most abundantly, but is now produced in bulk as a side product of the fermentation of *Streptomyces griseus* to obtain streptomycin. It is not synthesized by man who is dependent on natural sources and absorbs some 4–8 μg daily. Vitamin B_{12} (extrinsic factor) is normally well absorbed from the stomach in conjunction with intrinsic factor, a mucoprotein secreted by the gastrointestinal epithelium. The causes of failure to absorb vitamin B_{12} may be gastric as in pernicious anaemia or total gastrectomy; intestinal as in some diseases or surgical procedures in the ileum and (very rarely) the diet may be deficient as in the intake of vegans (vegetarians who eat no animal produce at all).

Pernicious anaemia. In this disease, vitamin B_{12} is not absorbed due to a deficiency of intrinsic factor and the typical set of findings include a histamine-fast gastric achlorhydria, a megaloblastic macrocytic anaemia and neurological signs of lesions of the posterolateral columns of the spinal cord (subacute combined degeneration). In the Schilling test, the alimentary absorption of the radioactive vitamin is determined by the measurement of the amount of uptake by the liver or excretion via the urine.

The symptoms can be reversed by the parenteral administration of vitamin B_{12} (Cyanocobalamin Injection B.P.) which will, however, not cure the disease and so must be continued for life. The correct diagnosis is therefore essential before treatment is begun. It is also important that folic acid is not used for though it improves the blood picture, it does not arrest and may indeed increase the neurological complications. The concurrent administration of iron may be needed due to the greatly accelerated erythropoiesis as shown by the increased reticulocyte count.

Hydroxocobalamin. This cobalamin derivative is more slowly absorbed than cyanocobalamin and more protein bound hence excretion is slow and higher blood levels result.

Folic acid (pteroyl monoglutamic acid)

This substance is a water-soluble vitamin found in green vegetables, yeast and liver. It plays an essential part in the formation of purine rings and some amino acids and is therefore important in nucleic acid synthesis and cell division. The normal adult requirement is approximately 50–70 μg daily, and the average British diet contains little surplus. It is normally well absorbed and converted in the body by folate reductase to the active form, folinic acid (citrovorum factor, tetrahydropteroylglutamic acid).

Frank deficiency is rare though lesser degrees are common and give a megaloblastic anaemia which is not identical with Pernicious Anaemia. Deficiency may be caused by a defective diet, various nutritional and malabsorption states, and in pregnancy where the need for folic acid rises sharply. Various drugs affect the metabolism of folic acid, perhaps by blocking folate reductase or by enhancing folic acid metabolism by enzyme induction, and a megaloblastic anaemia results. These drugs include phenytoin, primidone, phenobarbitone and the antifolic drugs used in the

The Blood-clotting mechanism

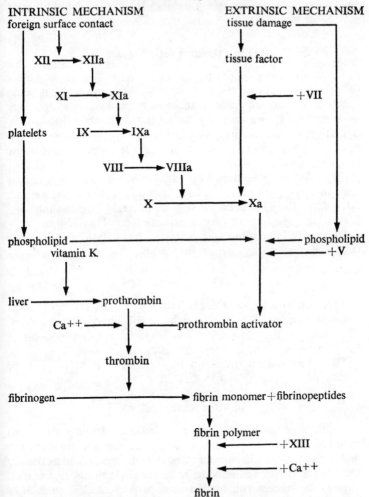

INTRINSIC MECHANISM
foreign surface contact

EXTRINSIC MECHANISM
tissue damage

XII → XIIa

tissue factor

XI → XIa

+VII

IX → IXa

VIII → VIIIa

platelets

X → Xa

phospholipid
vitamin K

phospholipid
+V

liver → prothrombin

Ca^{++} → ← prothrombin activator

thrombin

fibrinogen → fibrin monomer + fibrinopeptides

fibrin polymer
+XIII

+Ca^{++}

fibrin

The factors involved in the clotting of blood were assigned a Roman numeral by international agreement in 1957 to avoid confusion with the excess of synonyms previously prevailing.

This diagram shows the sequential theory of prothrombin activation where a cascade effect operates to convert a factor into the active enzyme which then acts on another factor and so on.

treatment of cancer. It is obviously of no use to give folic acid in these cases of drug-induced folic acid block though folinic acid may be of use.

Other Haemopoietic Factors

There are many other substances concerned in haemopoiesis though their exact function is disputed. Ascorbic acid has some functions in conjunction with those of cyanocobalamin and folic acid. Anaemia does occur in scurvy but there are other factors operating in this disease. Ascorbic acid may also be of use in iron deficiency anaemia as it will reduce ferric iron to the better absorbed ferrous form.

Other factors have been implicated in some forms of anaemia and include pyridoxine, cobalt, thyroxine, and testosterone. ACTH and the adrenocortical steroids not only suppress antibody formation and minimize the deleterious effects of antigen–antibody reactions as in autoimmune acquired haemolytic anaemia but may also cause some marrow stimulation.

ANTICOAGULANTS

Anticoagulant drugs are used to prevent extension of intravascular clotting and to diminish the likelihood of embolism. They are also used to prevent *in vitro* clotting to preserve blood for transfusion or laboratory examination.

The anticoagulant drugs act by interfering at some point or points in the pathway of blood clotting (see diagram above).

In Vitro Anticoagulants

Oxalic acid, sodium citrate and sodium edetate (see below) bind calcium and so prevent clotting. They are too toxic for use *in vivo* though sodium citrate is used in transfused blood as usually too little is introduced into the body for toxic effects to occur.

Heparin (discussed below) is used to prevent clotting *in vitro* and *in vivo* but anticoagulants such as the coumarins and the indanediones work only *in vivo*.

Sodium edetate. This drug chelates calcium, that is it forms a stable complex with the metal (cf. dimercaprol, page 171, and desferrioxamine mesylate, page 157). Sodium edetate is the sodium salt of ethylene diamine tetra-acetic acid (EDTA) which chelates alkaline earths in the descending order of preference, calcium, magnesium, potassium, sodium. The sodium–calcium complex of EDTA (sodium calciumedetate) chelates heavy metals and is used to treat lead poisoning as it mobilizes lead from the tissues and facilitates its excretion.

In Vivo Anticoagulants

1. Heparin

This naturally occurring substance is a complex mucopolysaccharide with a large number of sulphate groups. It was first isolated from the liver and is found especially in mast cells where granules give typical colour reactions.

Heparin acts *in vivo* and *in vitro* to prolong the clotting time and is thought to act by its strong electronegative charge interfering at several sites with the enzymes concerned in clotting. It inhibits the conversion of thrombin and fibrinogen to fibrin; of prothrombin to thrombin, and interferes with the clumping of platelets (i.e. thromboplastin generation). It also has lipolytic properties due to the activation of a lipoprotein lipase. Heparin is destroyed in the liver by the enzyme heparinase and is excreted via the urine.

Heparin is not effective orally and should be given intravenously when it acts almost at once to last for 4–6 hours. If given by the intramuscular or subcutaneous route, heparin may cause pain and bruising. The dosage of heparin is controlled by frequent measurement of the clotting time which is kept at 15–20 minutes (normal is 6–10 minutes). In therapy, however, the slower-acting oral anticoagulants (see below) are started at the same time as heparin which is discontinued when they have taken effect (in 24–36 hours).

There is an International Standard for heparin which contains either 118 or 130 units/mg, depending on the source, though in practice, it is convenient to assume that 1 mg contains 100 units.

The toxic effects of heparin, other than excessive anticoagulant effect, are few. They include hypersensitivity and alopecia.

Protamine sulphate. This substance will almost immediately reverse the action of heparin. It has strong electropositive charges which form an inactive complex with heparin though it has some anticoagulant properties of its own if given in excess. As a working approximation 1 mg of protamine sulphate is required for each 100 units (1 mg) of heparin.

2. The oral anticoagulants

These substances have no effect *in vitro* and do not act immediately *in vivo*. They reduce the formation of prothrombin, Factors VII, IX, and X in the liver perhaps by competition with vitamin K. The plasma prothrombin is decreased and the coagulation time increased but this effect is delayed in onset for the prothrombin already present has to be metabolized first. There are two major types of oral anticoagulant: the coumarin group and the indanedione group and administration is controlled by measuring the prothrombin time.

(a) *The coumarin group*. Warfarin (Warfarin Tablets B.P.) is typical of this group. It may also be given parenterally as it is water soluble. A therapeutic reduction of prothrombin occurs within 36 hours and the prothrombin time is back to normal within 3 days of stopping the drug. There are few toxic effects other than an occasional rash or dermatitis.

The older type of coumarin drug such as dicoumarol, ethyl biscoumacetate and cyclocoumarol are rarely used. More recent coumarin type drugs are phenprocoumon and nicoumalone.

(b) *The indanedione group*. Phenindione is typical of this group of oral anticoagulants (Phenindione Tablets B.P.). It has a rapid onset of action of short duration and there is a marked fall in prothrombin in 24 hours which reaches a therapeutic level in about 2 days. The prothrombin time returns to normal within 48–72 hours of stopping the drug.

It does have some serious toxic effects such as skin rashes, exfoliative dermatitis, renal damage, mouth ulcers, diarrhoea, leucopenia and jaundice though these occur in a very small percentage and at the beginning of treatment.

Vitamin K

The action of both the coumarins and the indanediones is reversed by the administration of vitamin K. This fat-soluble vitamin is essential for the synthesis of Factors VII, IX, and X which are concerned with blood clotting.

There are two natural forms of the vitamin: K_1 (phytomenadione) and K_2, both being naphthaquinone derivatives. Vitamin K is present in green leaves and fruit but is also synthesized by bacteria in the gut though probably absorbed only in the presence of bile salts.

Deficiency of the vitamin is not common but will cause haemorrhagic symptoms. It may result due to (i) reduced dietary intake, (ii) impairment of bacterial synthesis as in the administration of broad spectrum oral antibiotics or in neonates where the intestinal flora has not yet developed (haemorrhagic disease of the newborn), (iii) impaired absorption as in obstructive jaundice due to lack of bile salts or in the ingestion of large amounts of liquid paraffin which retains the vitamin.

Vitamin K is a specific antagonist of the coumarin or indanedione groups of anticoagulants, probably in a competitive fashion, and is used to counteract the haemorrhagic tendencies of overdosage. Phytomenadione Injection B.P. is a preparation of the natural vitamin and is the most rapidly acting preparation, taking only 3–5 hours to act. It is given intravenously or intramuscularly. The fat-soluble synthetic analogue Acetomenaphthone Tablets B.P. may be given orally but takes longer to act (24 hours) and is not absorbed in the absence of bile salts. Menadiol sodium diphosphate is a water-soluble analogue of vitamin K.

The interaction of other drugs with anticoagulants. The concurrent administration of some drugs can interfere with the action of anticoagulants. Oral antibiotics may decrease the endogenous production of vitamin K and salicylates act as weak competitive antagonists and so will reinforce the action of anticoagulants.

Chlorpromazine, phenylbutazone and clofibrate compete with anticoagulants for serum proteins. They will displace the anticoagulants and so raise the unbound (i.e. active) concentration.

Barbiturates, tranquillizers such as meprobamate and glutethimide cause enzyme induction (see page 13) which increases their metabolism and that of the warfarin-like drugs.

HYPOCHOLESTEROLAEMIC DRUGS

The plasma lipids consist of free fatty acids bound to albumin, and of triglycerides, phospholipids, free cholesterol and cholesterol esters mainly bound as lipoproteins characterized by their relative densities. Increase in plasma low density lipoproteins which contain some 60% of the plasma cholesterol as well as phospholipids and some triglycerides occurs in atherosclerosis though a causal relationship is not proven. Increases in very low density lipoproteins which contain mostly triglycerides occur in essential triglyceridaemia, diabetes and the nephrotic syndrome. Other patterns of increase in the plasma lipids also occur in a variety of diseases often of a familial nature.

Many drugs are capable of lowering the amounts of one or more of the plasma lipids but the evidence for their therapeutic value in the prevention of ischaemic heart disease or other complications is equivocal.

(i) *Cholestyramine*. This ion-exchange resin binds bile salts in the gut preventing their reabsorption by the enterohepatic circulation and subsequent use in cholesterol synthesis. This leads eventually to a fall in body cholesterol.

(ii) *Nicotinic acid*. This drug and some derivatives lowers plasma cholesterol but is likely to cause gastric upsets and flushing.

(iii) *Clofibrate*. This drug will reduce the plasma triglycerides and also plasma cholesterol but to a lesser degree. Its mode of action is not known but the effects produced are complex and include a rise in prothrombin time, a decrease in platelet stickiness, an increase in blood fibrinolytic activity and a decrease in blood fibrinogen. Although clofibrate appears of value in the long term treatment of ischaemic heart disease, its precise position is not known and the beneficial effects may be due to the actions other than the hypocholesterolaemic one.

(iv) *Other drugs*. Many drugs such as D-thyroxine, neomycin, oestrogens as well as the use of suitable diet will lower plasma lipid concentration.

FIBRINOLYSIS

Fibrin deposition can be due to clotting of the blood or to allergic, inflammatory and other trauma which allow plasma to leak into the tissues. These established thrombi are removed by a natural enzyme system in which the gamma globulin plasminogen is activated to plasmin which causes fibrinolysis. Plasmin is nor-

mally released in close proximity to the fibrin and is rapidly inactivated but if released in sufficient amounts in the plasma can
act on plasma proteins such as fibrinogen and other coagulation
factors to cause blood clotting defects.

Fibrinolysis is normally in equilibrium with clotting to maintain vascular patency and lyse unwanted fibrin. Fibrinolytic
therapy aims to accelerate the natural processes to restore vascular patency and several plasminogen activators are available. These
may be of use in deep venous thrombosis, pulmonary embolism,
myocardial infarction, peripheral or cerebral arterial occlusion.
They are best given by infusion as close as possible to the desired
site of action.

Streptokinase. This substance is an exotoxin derived from various strains of streptococcus. It is highly active as a plasminogen
activator but very antigenic.

Urokinase. This is derived from human urine but is so expensive
to isolate that use is unlikely to become widespread.

The therapeutic advantage of these plasminogen activators over
conventional anticoagulant therapy is that they do not rely merely
on preventing further clot and waiting for the long process of
natural recanalization but actively promote removal of the thrombosis. They are prone to cause further haemorrhage and their
place in therapy is as yet undecided.

Aminocaproic acid. This substance antagonizes the activation of
plasminogen and may be of use in hyperplasminaemic states such
as accidental or concealed haemorrhage in obstetrics and in lung
surgery.

Tranexamic acid. This is another antiplasmin substance.

Aprotinin. This substance has both antifibrinolytic and anti-
trypsin properties and can be used in acute pancreatitis.

REFERENCE
Biggs, R. (ed.) (1972) *Human Blood Coagulation, Haemostasis and
    Thrombosis*, Oxford: Blackwell Scientific.

14   The Kidney

PHYSIOLOGY OF THE KIDNEY

The ability of the kidney to modify the urine allows control of the overall concentration of body fluids, electrolytes and acid-base balance. The kidneys are also the chief organs of excretion of non-volatile substances.

Each kidney has about a million individual units called nephrons consisting of a glomerulus, proximal convoluted tubule, Loop of Henle, and distal convoluted tubule which leads into a collecting duct. Substances which reach the urine may be filtered at the glomerulus or secreted by the tubules, and their concentration in the urine will be the result of these processes and any reabsorption which may occur.

1. Glomerular Filtration

The glomerulus forms an almost protein-free filtrate virtually identical to plasma with respect to the diffusible constituents. The importance of adequate blood pressure and flow to the kidney is obvious, for these provide the operative force for the filtration which is essentially the same as at any other capillary bed though there are several differences as the efferent vessel is an arteriole, not a venule, and non-reabsorbed transudate is excreted to the exterior.

2. Tubular Reabsorption

Reabsorption processes in the renal tubules are of the utmost importance as a volume equal to the whole of the extracellular fluid is filtered by the glomerulus in $1\frac{1}{2}$ hours of which 99% is reabsorbed in the tubules. Unlike glomerular filtration, tubular reabsorption is not a hydrostatic mechanism but due mainly to energy using active transport processes.

(a) Proximal tubule

Here the glomerular filtrate is isotonic with plasma and about 80% is absorbed. Some 60–80% of the filtered sodium is reabsorbed in the proximal tubules by an active process which works against an electrochemical gradient.

There is also passive reabsorption of anion such as chloride which passes, as it were, downhill along the electrochemical gradient set up by the sodium. The major part of the filtered potassium is also reabsorbed in the proximal tubules but may be exchanged in the distal tubules for sodium.

Active tubular reabsorption of glucose, amino acids, creatine, lactate, citrate, uric acid, ascorbic acid and other organic compounds occurs mainly in the proximal convoluted tubule.

The proximal tubules and nearly all the rest of the nephron, save the ascending limb of the Loop of Henle, the distal convoluted tubules and collecting ducts, have a high water permeability not influenced by vasopressin. The movement of water across them is entirely passive and dependent on net solute movement which provides an osmotic gradient between the tubular and peritubular fluids so that water tends to pass out of the tubules to restore equilibrium.

The carbonic anhydrase mechanism. Carbon dioxide in the tubule cells reacts with water under the influence of carbonic anhydrase to form carbonic acid which ionizes to give bicarbonate and hydrogen ions. The hydrogen ions are secreted into the tubules and combine there with filtered bicarbonate to make carbonic acid which breaks down to form carbon dioxide which is absorbed, and water which is excreted. This mechanism exchanges hydrogen ion for tubular sodium ion which is thereby conserved. Carbonic anhydrase may be inhibited by such drugs as acetazolamide (page 173).

(b) Loop of Henle

As the tubular fluid passes along the Loop of Henle it becomes more concentrated in the descending limb due to entry of sodium and loss of water to the hypertonic surroundings. It becomes more dilute as it passes up the ascending limb due to the active reabsorption of sodium, not to the addition of water, so hypotonic fluid relatively weak in sodium enters the distal convoluted tubules. This process may be explained by the Counter Current Multiplier System. The descending limb is freely permeable to water but the ascending limb is not. As sodium is actively reabsorbed in the ascending limb, followed passively by such anions as chloride, the interstitial osmotic pressure of the renal medulla, into which the Loops of Henle dip, rises markedly. Most of the reabsorbed sodium passes back into the descending limb to enter the 'counter current' again and so maintains the hyperosmoticity of the peritubular tissue around the Loop of Henle. This hyperosmoticity is aided by the avascularity of the area which makes it less likely that ions will be carried away in the blood stream. The hyperosmoticity also increases progressively as the medulla descends towards the renal papillae and reaches a maximum at the papillary tips. The importance of the multiplier system is that the collecting ducts also pass through the hyperosmotic pertubular tissue (see below).

(c) The distal convoluted tubules

In the distal convoluted tubules, salts, together with an osmotic equivalent of water (provided body hydration is normal), are absorbed into the peritubular tissue and rapidly dissipate because of the very good blood supply. Therefore the tubular fluid delivered to the collecting ducts is of decreased volume but similar tonicity to that which arrived from the Loop of Henle. Sodium is not only actively reabsorbed in the distal convoluted tubules but is also reabsorbed by exchange for potassium and hydrogen ion. The excretion of potassium will increase if the sodium is accompanied by a non-diffusible ion rather than by the freely diffusible chloride as sodium can then be reabsorbed only by ion exchange.

(d) The collecting ducts

These traverse the region of hypertonic peritubular fluid around the Loops of Henle and with the distal convoluted tubules are impermeable to water save if under the influence of vasopressin (page 105). If vasopressin is present, water will be absorbed and a urine formed which is isotonic with the interstitial fluid and so hypertonic to plasma.

Up to four-fifths of the tubular fluid leaving the ascending limb is reabsorbed in the distal nephron and the rest may be concentrated up to five times in the collecting ducts without destroying the hypertonicity of the peritubular fluids.

In the absence of vasopressin the absorption of salt can still take place but water cannot follow and a large amount of hypotonic urine is formed. In diabetes insipidus the normal secretion of vasopressin fails and large amounts of urine are excreted daily equivalent to that amount of tubular fluid leaving the distal convoluted tubules (perhaps as much as 20 litres).

3. Tubular Secretion

Some compounds are actively secreted into the urine by the kidney tubules. There are two main mechanisms; one for the transport of organic acids and another for organic bases.

Acidic drugs are those which donate hydrogen ions and include phenobarbitone, salicylates, penicillin, the sulphonamides. Basic drugs combine with hydrogen ions and include amphetamine, imipramine, mecamylamine, pempidine, pethidine and quinidine.

Whilst some compounds may be actively secreted, they may also be passively absorbed at a rate which depends on the concentration gradient, their lipid solubility, degree of ionization and the urinary pH. Hence their final concentration in the urine depends on the balance of these factors which are further discussed on page 177.

DIURETICS

A diuretic is a substance that increases the excretion of urine. This definition would therefore include water, the physiological diuretic, but clinically it is customary to restrict the term to substances which cause a net loss of sodium and water from the body and to exclude such substances as water, digitalis and alcohol.

In many pathological conditions there is a progressive impairment of the ability of the kidney to excrete excess sodium. This retention of sodium results in oedema due to the increased extracellular fluid needed to contain it. The aim of diuretic therapy is to increase the net loss of sodium to facilitate the contraction of this pathologically large extracellular space.

It is possible to increase the formation of urine (and so sodium excretion) by increasing glomerular filtration, diminishing tubular reabsorption or by increasing tubular secretion, though in practice only the first two mechanisms are important.

1. Osmotic diuretics

Any increase in the solute excreted in the urine means that the output of water will rise as the kidney is capable of only a limited amount of osmotic work in concentrating the urine. This diuresis is independent of vasopressin levels as the only function of this hormone is to make the wall of the collecting ducts permeable to water.

(a) *Sodium sulphate*. Sulphate is an indiffusible ion and, after glomerular filtration, remains in the tubules increasing the osmoticity and hence the urine flow. On reaching the distal tubule, due to a lack of diffusible anion, such as chloride, the exchange mechanism of potassium for sodium will predominate and there will be increased potassium loss in the urine (page 168).

(b) *Glucose*. In diabetes mellitus the plasma level of glucose may rise above the renal threshold. Glucose will then appear in the urine and act as an osmotic diuretic.

2. Mercurial diuretics

Soluble compounds of mercury which produce mercuric ion act as diuretics though only the organic mercurials are used in therapy as the inorganic compounds are too toxic.

The mercurial diuretics are poorly absorbed by mouth and are usually given by injection. They are plasma bound but concentrate in the renal cortex and are secreted into the urine as cysteine complexes. Some may pass into the bile and cause gastrointestinal symptoms.

The mercurial diuretics inhibit the absorption of sodium in the proximal renal tubules by releasing mercuric ions which form inactive mercaptide complexes with sulphydryl (-SH) containing enzymes vital for electrolyte transport. This action on the enzymes is antagonized by thiol or dithiol compounds such as dimercaprol (BAL, British Anti-Lewisite), which is discussed below.

In the distal tubules a lot of this excess sodium is exchanged for potassium and hydrogen ion but little chloride is reabsorbed. This results in a large volume of urine with more chloride than sodium and containing increased hydrogen ion and potassium. This may eventually cause a hypochloraemic metabolic alkalosis.

The diuretic response lessens after a few doses of the mercurial as its dissociation into mercuric ions is reduced by the alkalosis. However, acidifying salts such as ammonium chloride reduce the pH and facilitate the production of mercuric ions and allow the diuresis to continue. Carbonic anhydrase inhibitors also potentiate the diuretic action of the organic mercurials (page 172).

Mersalyl. This organic mercurial has been replaced today by the potent oral diuretics such as frusemide (page 174). Injection of Mersalyl B.P. contains 10% of the sodium salt of mersalyl acid and 5% of theophylline. The theophylline does have an appreciable effect by increasing the free water clearance, and also allowing the mercurial complex to be better absorbed. Mersalyl is given intramuscularly as subcutaneous injection may cause tissue necrosis, and intravenous injection may cause arrhythmias such as ventricular fibrillation. Other toxic effects are hypersensitivity, allergic rashes, renal damage, and chronic mercury poisoning (as 1 ml of Mersalyl Injection contains 40 mg of mercury).

Mersalyl causes a diuresis in 3 hours which is maximal in 7 hours and lasts for 24 hours. It is given 2–3 times a week, preceded by ammonium chloride.

Dimercaprol (British Anti-Lewisite, BAL). This compound competes with the tissue –SH groups for mercury (and other heavy metals such as arsenic, gold, antimony, bismuth but not lead or iron) to form an inactive complex with the metal which is excreted via the urine.

Dimercaprol is given intramuscularly and may produce nausea, vomiting, lachrimation and salivation. It was originally developed as an antidote to the poisonous arsenic gas, lewisite.

3. The acidifying diuretics

Ammonium chloride, if taken by mouth, is nauseating and irritant to the stomach but may be given as enteric coated tablets which do not release the drug till the intestine is reached.

On absorption, ammonium chloride is ionized to ammonium

and chloride ions. The ammonium is metabolized to urea by the liver and this urea is excreted by the kidney and acts as a weak osmotic diuretic. The reaction further yields hydrogen ions which have an acidifying action on the blood and urine to cause a metabolic acidosis. The excess chloride ion is excreted by the kidney accompanied by an equivalent amount of cation which is mainly sodium and some potassium. There is also an iso-osmotic amount of water.

After a lag phase of a few days, however, the kidney forms ammonia from glutamate and this is used to neutralize excess chloride so sodium is no longer excreted to act as a diuretic.

4. The xanthine diuretics (see page 222)

Caffeine, theobromine and theophylline have weak diuretic actions. They have a haemodynamic effect increasing the cardiac output and the renal blood flow which increases glomerular filtration. The xanthines also inhibit the reabsorption of sodium and chloride from the renal tubules.

Theophylline (as Aminophylline Injection B.P.) is the most commonly used. Theophylline is also a component of Mersalyl Injection B.P.

5. The carbonic anhydrase inhibitors

The carbonic anhydrase mechanism (page 167) allows the kidney to conserve sodium and to secrete an acid urine. Some drugs inhibit carbonic anhydrase and was first noticed in sulphanilamide.

Inhibition of carbonic anhydrase means that less hydrogen ion enters the tubules and therefore will not be available for exchange with sodium which will however still exchange with potassium whose loss in the urine increases. The net result is the production of large volumes of alkaline urine containing much sodium and potassium, and a metabolic acidosis caused by the retention of hydrogen ion and the loss of bicarbonate. There may also be a hypokalaemia due to the increased loss of potassium.

The response to carbonic anhydrase inhibitors decreases rapidly perhaps because in acidosis there are sufficient hydrogen ions to operate the cation exchange process even without carbonic anhydrase. More carbon dioxide is also given off in the lungs to compensate for the acidosis so the plasma bicarbonate falls and its loss in the urine decreases.

The therapeutically useful carbonic anhydrase inhibitors such as acetazolamide and dichlorphenamide are little used as diuretics alone. They may be used alternately with mercurial diuretics which cause a metabolic alkalosis and so will potentiate the action of the carbonic anhydrase inhibitors.

The inhibition of carbonic anhydrase will lessen the secretion of aqueous humour and so may be used to treat glaucoma. These drugs also have a place in the treatment of epilepsy (page 204).

6. The thiadiazines (thiazides)

Chlorothiazide is the parent compound of a group of orally effective diuretics, the thiadiazines, which are heterocyclic sulphonamides in structure. They are weak carbonic anhydrase inhibitors and depress the tubular reabsorption of sodium and chloride. The inhibition of carbonic anhydrase causes potassium depletion and it may be advisable to give potassium supplements. This depletion, which may be severe enough to cause a hypokalaemic alkalosis, is of especial importance when digitalis is also being used.

Chlorothiazide is poorly absorbed by mouth but may be used orally. More recent thiadiazine derivatives such as hydrochlorothiazide, hydroflumethiazide and bendrofluazide are generally more potent than chlorothiazide on a weight for weight basis though they do not appear to be less toxic. A single morning dose of a thiadiazine is usually sufficient.

The thiadiazine diuretics have a variety of other actions of which one, an antihypertensive effect, is of clinical use. Although sodium depletion lowers the blood pressure by loss of extracellular fluid, the thiadiazines appear to have a direct action on the blood vessels as well and may reduce the vasoconstrictor action of noradrenaline. Evidence for a direct action came from a related substance, diazoxide, which retains sodium, is not diuretic, yet will still lower blood pressure. Diazoxide may be used clinically for its hypotensive effect (page 152), or to raise blood glucose (page 120). The hypotensive action of the thiadiazines is also maintained despite deliberate correction of the plasma volume and electrolyte loss and, even without deliberate correction, these levels tend to return spontaneously to the pretreatment levels.

Paradoxically, the thiadiazines may be of use in the treatment of diabetes insipidus and decrease the volume of urine by 50% but the mechanism is not known. They also have various metabolic effects and may aggravate diabetes mellitus by a direct depression of the pancreatic β cells. This diabetogenic tendency occurs especially on long-term therapy and is usually reversible on withdrawal of the drug. The plasma uric acid may rise but usually causes no symptoms though attacks of gout sometimes occur. Other toxic effects are rare but include skin rashes, thrombocytopenic purpura and, very rarely, more serious blood dyscrasias.

Clorexolone. Clorexolone has a chemical structure similar to that of hydrochlorothiazide but has a different heterocyclic ring. It is about twenty times as potent on a weight for weight basis and, taken orally, causes a diuresis which is maximal in 2–4 hours and lasts 12–48 hours.

7. Frusemide

This is a non-mercurial diuretic, chemically distinct from the thiadiazines but related as it has a similar halogenated sulphamoyl benzene ring. Frusemide inhibits the active reabsorption of sodium in the distal and proximal tubules but does not inhibit carbonic anhydrase.

On oral administration it causes a rapid diuresis which lasts for 4–6 hours. Intravenously, frusemide causes a torrential diuresis which could amount to a third of the glomerular filtrate and so could easily cause dehydration and circulatory collapse.

The major toxic effects of frusemide are the electrolyte disturbances secondary to the massive diuresis. The urinary loss of potassium is less than that of the thiadiazines but may still be a problem especially if hepatic disease is present. Frusemide can cause hyperuricaemia and disturbances in carbohydrate metabolism but this diabetogenic tendency is less than that of the thiadiazines.

Frusemide, perhaps, should be reserved for those occasions such as pulmonary oedema or acute congestive cardiac failure when there is extreme haste.

8. Ethacrynic acid

Ethacrynic acid is a phenoxyacetic acid derivative and has no structural relationship to the thiadiazine or mercurial diuretics. It probably affects the ascending limb of the Loop of Henle and blocks sodium and chloride reabsorption in the proximal and distal tubules. Potassium excretion is increased and supplementary potassium may be necessary.

Ethacrynic acid is readily absorbed after oral administration to cause a diuresis in 30 minutes, maximal in 3–6 hours. Intravenously, ethacrynic acid is effective in a couple of minutes to cause a diuresis which is complete in 90 minutes.

The most serious side effects are the electrolyte disturbances caused by its powerful diuretic action which, like those of frusemide, can cause hypotension and circulatory collapse.

9. Triamterene

Triamterene is a pteridine compound which increases the excretion of sodium, bicarbonate and water but depresses the excretion of potassium. It is not an aldosterone antagonist as was once thought but does have similar actions. Triamterene acts directly on the distal tubules to depress the reabsorption of sodium and the exchange of sodium for potassium. There is no carbonic anhydrase inhibition and the excretion of uric acid rises.

Triamterene is not a powerful diuretic compared with the thiadiazines, frusemide or ethacrynic acid but the properties of diminishing potassium loss and increasing the excretion of uric acid can be an advantage. It is usually given with other drugs such as the thiazides.

10. Amiloride

This substance has similar actions to triamterene but is more powerful as a diuretic. It will prevent the net potassium loss of even such vigorous oral diuretics as ethacrynic acid and frusemide.

11. Aldosterone antagonists

Aldosterone (page 107) increases the reabsorption of sodium and chloride by the distal convoluted tubules and decreases their loss in the sweat and the gut. It also increases the exchange of potassium for sodium in the kidney tubules.

Spironolactone. This has a structure similar to that of aldosterone and acts as a competitive antagonist thus promoting renal loss of sodium and retention of potassium. Spironolactone is effective only when there is an increase in the amount of sodium delivered to the distal tubules so it is necessary to use it in combination with other diuretics, such as the thiadiazines, which act proximally on sodium reabsorption. Spironolactone is cumulative in action and the full response may not be seen for some days.

There are few side effects but spironolactone should be used only in cases where there is an excess of aldosterone such as in hepatic cirrhosis or thrombosis of the inferior vena cava.

Diuretics and potassium

The daily intake of potassium in a good mixed diet is about 60–80 mEq and is ample to supply the normal basic daily need of 20–30 mEq. Many diuretics tend to deplete potassium in the body, though triamterene, amiloride and spironolactone tend to conserve potassium. Diuretics causing potassium loss include the mercurial diuretics, the carbonic anhydrase inhibitors, the thiadiazines, frusemide and ethacrynic acid. The normal dietary intake of potassium is not always sufficient to guard against deficiency in a patient on these diuretics especially if therapy is prolonged.

Potassium depletion causes lethargy, muscular weakness, a low T wave in the ECG and increased sensitivity to digitalis. It may be associated with chloride depletion and a metabolic alkalosis. There are several methods of administering potassium supplements and the need is for about 20–40 mEq daily.

(a) *Fresh fruit juice* (but not squash). Oranges and grape fruit contain a lot of potassium, but as one pound of fresh oranges contains only 12–14 mEq of potassium, a lot may have to be eaten daily, which is expensive, time consuming, and could be nauseating.

(b) *Potassium chloride.* 0·5 g tablets of Potassium Chloride Tablets B.P. contain 6·5 mEq but may cause severe gastric irritation. There are enteric coated forms which may be passed entire or cause ulceration of the intestine. Slow-K is a proprietary brand of slow release potassium chloride (600 mg) and patients may be able to tolerate it.

(c) *Potassium Effervescent Tablets* B.P.C. These contain 6·5 mEq of potassium and are more palatable but do not supply chloride ion and hence do not correct any accompanying alkalosis. It may, indeed, be difficult to supply chloride if the patient is on a salt-restricted diet.

Alteration of urine pH

It is often desirable to alter the pH of the urine. This is normally about pH 6, though becomes more acid on a protein diet or if concentrated. A vegetarian diet tends to cause an alkaline urine.

Alteration of the pH of the urine may be necessary to provide a suitable environment for drugs to work, such as the urinary antiseptics. Diuretics such as mersalyl are potentiated in an acid urine.

A more recent use of changing urinary pH is to control the excretion of drugs. When a neutral un-ionized drug passes into the renal tubules after glomerular filtration, it will be rapidly reabsorbed as it is lipid soluble. The ionized drug, on the other hand, is poorly absorbed from the renal tubules and so excretion will be high. The degree of ionization depends on the pH of the urine and basic drugs (such as amphetamine or pethidine) are greatly ionized in acid urine, whereas acidic drugs (such as phenobarbitone or salicylate) are more ionized in alkaline urine. The relevance to treatment of poisoning by these drugs is obvious.

The urine may be made alkaline by potassium or sodium citrate as the citrate is metabolized leaving excess of the cation. Sodium bicarbonate may be used but has the disadvantage of releasing carbon dioxide in the stomach when taken orally.

Acidification of the urine is usually achieved by ammonium chloride (page 171). A ketogenic diet, ascorbic acid, methionine or arginine will also lower urine pH.

URIC ACID METABOLISM AND GOUT

Uric acid is the main end product of purine metabolism in man and is excreted via the kidneys. Hyperuricaemia (not always associated with the clinical sydnrome of gout) may result from excessive production or defective excretion of uric acid.

Excessive production may result from an inborn error of metabolism or some cases of myelo-proliferative disease. Hyperuricaemia may also be of iatrogenic origin due to such drugs as acetazolamide, the thiadiazines, low doses of salicylates, and is perhaps due to interference with renal excretion.

The symptoms of gout result from the crystal deposition of uric acid and prolonged hyperuricaemia. These may cause an acute or chronic arthritis, gouty nephropathy and vascular disease. Two groups of drugs are available to treat gout: those acting symptomatically and those acting metabolically.

1. Symptomatic Drugs

(i) *Colchicine*. This is a substance obtained from the autumn crocus (*Colchicum autumnale*). It specifically relieves the pain of acute gout and no other type of arthritis. Its mode of action is ill understood and it has no effect on serum uric acid levels and does not seem to promote renal excretion of uric acid.

Colchicine is a toxic drug causing renal damage and gastroenteritis. It also has an antimitotic action and will arrest cell division in the metaphase; an action which has been the subject of much experimental work.

(ii) *Indomethacin*; *phenylbutazone*; *corticosteroids*. These drugs are discussed elsewhere.

2. Metabolic Drugs

These may be uricosuric drugs which interfere with the renal tubular reabsorption of uric acid and so promote its excretion or they may be xanthine oxidase inhibitors which lessen the production of uric acid.

(a) *Uricosuric drugs*. Uric acid excretion is influenced by a large number of drugs which seem to be excreted by the same transport system in the renal tubules. These drugs include penicillin, probenecid, hippuric acid, phenol red, and some agents, such as diodrast, which are used in X-ray contrast techniques. Most uricosuric drugs increase the clearance of uric acid when given in high doses but may decrease it in low doses. The blood level of

THE KIDNEY 179

uric acid in gout may take some time to fall due to the enormous tissue reservoir. The excretion may also be so high that crystallization of uric acid occurs in the renal tract. This crystallization may be avoided by alkalization of the urine and a high fluid output.

(i) Aspirin. This is uricosuric in high doses only and may block the uricosuric action of other drugs such as probenecid (page 263).

(ii) Probenecid. This is a long-established uricosuric drug and inhibits the renal tubular transport of organic acids including penicillin.

(iii) Sulphinpyrazone. This drug is a congener of phenylbutazone and is a potent inhibitor of renal tubular reabsorption of uric acid. It is more toxic than probenecid.

(b) *Xanthine oxidase inhibitors*. These drugs reduce the formation of uric acid from purines by inhibiting the enzyme xanthine oxidase. The oxypurines, hypoxanthine and xanthine, are excreted instead and, as they are soluble, do not present the same problem. Allopurinol is a therapeutically useful xanthine oxidase inhibitor. It is readily absorbed and troublesome side effects are not common.

REFERENCES

Berliner, K. H. & Baer, J. E. (1961) Physiological basis for the action of newer diuretic agents. *Pharmacological Reviews*, **13**, 517.

Goldberg, M. (1967) The physiology and pathophysiology of diuretic agents. In *Modern Trends in Pharmacology and Therapeutics*, W. F. M. Fulton (ed.) **1**, 41. London: Butterworth.

Heller, H. & Ginsburg, M. (1961) Diuretic drugs. In *Progress in Medicinal Chemistry*, **1**, 132. Ellis, G. P. & West, G. B. (eds.) London: Butterworth.

15   The Central Nervous System I

ANALGESIC DRUGS

An analgesic drug abolishes the appreciation of pain but not environmental and sensory perception (Gk *an*, not; *algeo*, to free pain). This is in contrast to the general anaesthetics which abolish both pain and perception of the environment. A narcotic analgesic produces both analgesia and depression of the central nervous system (Gk. *narkosis*, a benumbing).

Knowledge of the mechanism of pain is incomplete but it is unlikely to be a specific modality with sequential afferent conduction to a 'pain centre'. Whilst not universally accepted, the recently proposed Gate Control Theory allows a better understanding of the variations in the individual response to pain. The theory proposes that the substantia gelatinosa acts as a gate to impulses from the periphery and may or may not be open to allow onward transmission to higher centres. A 'central control trigger' makes the decision to allow afferent stimuli to pass the gate based on such factors as emotion, past experience and present circumstances. The impulses then pass to an 'action system' which brings into play the appropriate response to the pain stimulus.

Pain may be of paramount diagnostic importance and its uncritical relief before making a correct diagnosis could be disastrous. It may be relieved in two ways. The cause of the pain may be removed or its central appreciation altered. The central appreciation of pain may be changed either at a low level (the perception of pain); or at the cortical level (the emotional reaction to pain). Pain may also be relieved by the use of local analgesics (see page 240) which prevent the sensation of pain from a region of the body reaching the central nervous system.

The ideal analgesic. This would act only on the lower central perception of pain, but all the potent drugs so far known act both at this level and the cortex. It is perhaps this cortical action which makes the powerful analgesics the cause of drug dependence. The ideal analgesic would also have other properties such as producing satisfactory analgesia over wide ranges of pain on either oral or parenteral administration and be useful regardless of age or disease. It should have minimal side effects especially on the respiration, circulation and cerebration whether the patient be ambulant or not.

All new analgesics should be considered under these headings and compared with morphine which is the standard powerful analgesic.

The laboratory testing of new analgesics is extremely difficult, though may act as a guide and reveal toxic effects. The usual experimental methods of producing pain are by thermal or electrical stimulation; by mechanical pressure; by the injection of irritants, and by ischaemia.

Clinical testing is also very difficult but the final test of any new analgesic is its power to safely relieve pain associated with disease in man. In clinical testing it is usually the subjective rather than the quantitative relief of pain that is measured and due allowance must be made for subjective factors such as placebo effect, observer error and for variations in the clinical course of the disease.

Analgesics are commonly considered under the headings of the powerful (or narcotic) analgesics such as morphine, and the mild (or antipyretic) analgesics such as aspirin. There are some drugs which relieve specific pains only and have no analgesic action otherwise. An example of this type of drug is colchicine, which relieves the pain of gout but not other pain (page 178).

POWERFUL (NARCOTIC) ANALGESICS

Opium

Opium is the dried latex obtained by incising the unripe capsule of the opium poppy (*Papaver somniferum*). It contains two chemical types of active constituents: the phenanthrene derivatives such as morphine, codeine, and thebaine; and the isoquinoline derivatives such as papaverine and narcotine. Papaverine is not a narcotic but a smooth muscle relaxant (page 148).

The value of opium as a powerful analgesic was known by the time of the earliest written records, but it is rarely used nowadays in crude form. Papaveretum is a mixture of the pure alkaloids and is sometimes used but, as its main active constituent is morphine (50%), the side effects are not less than those of morphine.

Morphine

This drug is the standard powerful analgesic and forms some 10% of crude opium. Morphine is absorbed from the gut, but this may be slow and erratic and it is usually given subcutaneously or intramuscularly and acts in 15 minutes to give analgesia for 4–6 hours.

Morphine is distributed widely and is biotransformed in the liver. It is mainly excreted in the urine as the bound form, conjugated with glucuronic acid, though some is excreted in the faeces, sweat, bile, gastric juice and milk. Morphine will also cross the placenta and its use in obstetrical analgesia must take into account the potential respiratory depressant effects on the fetus.

The basic action of morphine is little understood but it does block release of acetylcholine and the action of 5-hydroxytryptamine at some peripheral sites. These substances are thought to be central transmitters and at least some of the actions of morphine can be explained by their inhibition. Morphine analgesia seems to be a combination of several discrete mechanisms including elevation of pain threshold, alteration in response to pain stimuli and induction of sleep. There is a change in affective response rather than a reduction of pain perception but other sensory modalities appear not to be affected. It is possible that drugs like morphine influence the descending pathways of the central control trigger blocking the passage of a potential pain stimulus (see page 180).

The pharmacological actions of morphine

(a) *The central nervous system.* Morphine depresses the central nervous system but also has some primary excitatory effects.

Morphine in small doses (say 10 mg in an adult) gives analgesia with no marked hypnotic effect and associated with a sense of detachment, relaxation, tranquillity and increased ability to tolerate pain and discomfort (euphoria). Larger doses produce both analgesia and sleep. Morphine produces analgesia especially of severe and continuous pain of the visceral type and probably acts by a cortical effect to depress the appreciation of pain.

Morphine selectively depresses the respiratory centre by lowering the sensitivity of the centre to rises in Pco_2. This depression is proportional to dose and may make morphine unsuitable for patients with pulmonary disease. Morphine passes the placenta so, if given in labour, can depress the respiration of the new-born child. Morphine may also cause release of histamine and 5-hydroxytryptamine and these, by bronchoconstriction, contribute further to the respiratory depression. Morphine also depresses the cough centre and some related compounds such as codeine are much used for their anti-tussive (anti-cough) action.

Morphine has several excitatory effects. It will cause nausea and vomiting, especially in the ambulant patient, due to a central action upon the emetic chemoreceptor zone with perhaps some vestibular stimulation, but it does not act on the vomiting centre itself. Morphine has a convulsant action and should not be used to control convulsions from other causes. Morphine also causes constriction of the pupil probably by stimulation of the third nerve nucleus.

(b) *Smooth muscle*. Morphine acts directly on smooth muscle to reduce motility and increase tone. Intestinal passage time is prolonged to cause constipation made worse by the central action of morphine lessening the desire to defaecate. This constipating effect may be very troublesome when morphine is used as an analgesic, but is sometimes used to control diarrhoea. There is also some biliary tract spasm and the relief by morphine of the pain of biliary colic is entirely central. The tone of the ureter and bladder sphincter is also increased.

(c) *Cardiovascular system*. Morphine has very little effect on the circulatory system in therapeutic doses though there may be some postural hypotension due to peripheral vasodilatation caused by vasomotor centre depression and the liberation of histamine. The release of histamine may also cause a Triple Response at the site of injection. The peripheral vasodilatation caused by morphine may be associated with sweating and produce a fall in body temperature.

The uses and limitations of morphine

Morphine is used mainly to relieve severe pain and to sedate and allay anxiety in shock. It is also used to control diarrhoea; as part of the treatment of paroxysmal noctural dyspnoea; and as a premedication before operative surgery.

Most of the side effects of morphine have already been mentioned. These include nausea and vomiting (especially in the ambulant patient) and constipation. Depression of respiration can be marked and large doses of morphine may kill by stopping the breathing altogether.

Morphine is a drug which can cause dependence and tolerance even after a few hours of use. This is an extremely important property of the opium analgesics and their synthetic substitutes and is discussed on page 237.

Morphine antagonists

Overdose of morphine may result from such circumstances as mistake; suicidal intent; or by transmission across the placenta which affects the fetus. Morphine and related compounds are specifically antagonized by such compounds as nalorphine, levallorphan or naloxone (page 185) so analeptics (page 221) are not needed to stimulate the central nervous system depressed by morphine and may even be hazardous as they may synergize with the convulsant action of morphine. The mode of action of these narcotic antagonists is not fully understood and theories involving simple competitive antagonism (see pp. 22, 23) at a single receptor do not fully explain the findings. Some of the antagonists also have actions like morphine (i.e. agonist actions) as well as the antagonist actions. Nalorphine, for example, will reverse the respiratory depression produced by morphine but can also produce respiratory depression itself. On the other hand naloxone has virtually pure antagonist actions with little or no agonist action.

It may be that these drugs have their effects at different groups of receptors in the central nervous system called the morphine (M) and nalorphine (N) receptors and differences in affinity and activity at these receptors account for the variable picture. Morphine has a high affinity and activity at the M receptor but little effect at the N receptor. Nalorphine has a high affinity for the M receptor but little activity there and would antagonize the action of morphine. Nalorphine also has a high affinity and activity in the N receptor and thus can produce analgesia, respiratory depression and other agonist actions. Naloxone has a high affinity for both types of receptors but very little intrinsic activity and is thus a pure antagonist.

The narcotic antagonists are used to treat overdose of morphine-like drugs, including pethidine, when they rapidly reverse the respiratory and circulatory depression. They will also induce withdrawal symptoms in a person dependent on the morphine-like drugs. It is very important to realize that the narcotic antagonists will not reverse the depression caused by other drugs such as alcohol or the barbiturates and indeed this could be worsened by the agonist actions of nalorphine.

(a) *Nalorphine.* Nalorphine (*N*-allylnormorphine) is closely related to morphine and differs only in the replacement of a methyl group by an allyl group and has similar but weaker effects. It is not used as an analgesic in man as it causes feelings of tension and even hallucinations.

Nalorphine has an action lasting 2–3 hours so may need to be repeated in the treatment of morphine poisoning as the action of morphine lasts some 6 hours. Nalorphine, unlike naloxone, does not antagonize the actions of pentazocine.

(b) *Levallorphan.* This drug bears the same relationship to levorphanol (page 188) as nalorphine does to morphine. It is also a competitive antagonist of the morphine-like drugs.

(c) *Pentazocine.* This narcotic antagonist is discussed on page 188.

(d) *Naloxone* (*N*-allylnoroxymorphone). This drug is a powerful narcotic antagonist devoid of agonist action. It is the drug of choice in morphine overdose and unlike nalorphine, will also antagonize the action of pentazocine.

Other Powerful Analgesics

Morphine has a great many defects, so much effort has gone into the search for a suitable substitute and there is available a vast number of synthetic drugs as well as other compounds isolated from opium.

It is thought by many that potent analgesic action is closely linked to the dependence-causing and respiratory-depressant properties of morphine derivatives but drugs such as nalorphine, which antagonize the actions of morphine-like analgesics are themselves analgesic but have a low dependence producing potential. Unfortunately the unpleasant feelings produced by nalorphine precludes its use as an analgesic but newer antagonists such as pentazocine are clinically useful. It is advisable to approach all claims that a new drug is THE substitute for morphine with cautious cynicism until extended trials have shown its worth.

Morphine derivatives

1. *Codeine.* Codeine is methyl morphine and occurs naturally in opium (0·5%). It is much less analgesic than morphine and the maximum analgesia possible is about ¼–1/10th of morphine. It is inadequate for severe pain as large doses are prone to cause excitement and vomiting.

Codeine may be given on its own, usually as the phosphate (Codeine Phosphate Tablets B.P.), or in combination with other drugs such as aspirin. Aspirin, Phenacetin and Codeine Tablets B.P. (codeine compound tablets) contain 250 mg each of aspirin and phenacetin and 8 mg of codeine phosphate.

Codeine is well absorbed from the gut and is used especially as an antitussive (Codeine Linctus B.P.C.); an analgesic, and an antidiarrhoeal drug. It is practically devoid of psychic action and in practice is not a drug of dependence.

2. *Dihydrocodeine.* This drug is a semi-synthetic derivative of codeine. It is a mild analgesic similar to codeine but may have less side effects, and is suitable for ambulant patients with mild pain.

3. *Diamorphine hydrochloride (diacetyl morphine, heroin).* Diamorphine is a semi-synthetic derivative of morphine in which both hydroxyl groups have been acetylated. It causes similar analgesia and respiratory depression to morphine but less nausea, vomiting, constipation and sedation. The analgesic action of diamorphine is more rapid of onset than morphine but lasts 2–3 hours only.

Diamorphine is very prone to cause dependence and its use is illegal in many countries.

4. *Pholcodine.* This drug is the morpholinoethyl ether of morphine and is used for its cough depressant activity. It is less toxic than codeine.

5. *Apomorphine.* Like morphine, apomorphine stimulates the emetic chemoreceptor zone but this action is much enhanced and the analgesic properties are abolished. Apomorphine may be used to induce vomiting in patients who have ingested poison but is too drastic in action and other methods of treatment are preferable.

Apomorphine is used by psychiatrists in aversion therapy to treat alcoholism or homosexuality, when a strong dislike may be induced by using Pavlovian principles of the conditioned reflex.

Synthetic drugs with a morphine-like action

1. *Pethidine (meperidine) and other piperidine derivatives.* Pethidine is a synthetic drug unrelated to morphine and was found in a search for a spasmolytic drug with atropine-like properties.

It may be given orally or by injection and acts in a few minutes for 3–4 hours and is metabolized mainly in the liver. The maximum analgesic effect possible is greater than that of codeine but less than that of morphine, and 100 mg of pethidine causes similar analgesia to 10 mg morphine. In equianalgesic doses, morphine and pethidine probably cause the same degree of respiratory depression. Pethidine does not usefully suppress cough.

Large doses of pethidine may cause tremors and convulsions. It is not constipating but will cause smooth muscle spasm and its atropine-like action is of little importance save in the production of some side effects, which include sweating, nausea, thirst, dry mouth and dizziness. Tolerance and dependence can develop and its actions are antagonized by drugs such as nalorphine. Other piperidine derivatives such as phenoperidine and fentanyl are used mainly in anaesthetic practise (see 'neuroleptanalgesia' page 220). They are of extreme potency on a weight for weight basis but in equianalgesic doses produce the same degree of respiratory depression as morphine. They are, however, largely devoid of hypnotic and sedative properties, provide good cardiovascular stability and are less emetic than morphine. Given intravenously they have a rapid onset of action which is of short duration (one hour for phenoperidine and 20–30 minutes for fentanyl).

2. *Methadone group.* Methadone (amidone) produces similar analgesia and respiratory depression to morphine though structurally it is only remotely related. It has a longer duration of action and is reliably absorbed by mouth. Methadone can cause nausea, dizziness and a dry mouth especially in the ambulant patient. Dependence does occur though is less severe than with morphine or heroin and methadone is often used in substitution therapy in the treatment of opiate dependence. Dextropropoxyphene is also a member of the methadone group though is far less potent and is similar to codeine.

3. *Pentazocine.* This analgesic is a member of the benzomorphan group which also includes phenazocine. Pentazocine is a relatively weak narcotic antagonist i.e. it will block the agonist actions of morphine but also has marked agonist actions of its own. It can produce analgesia comparable to that of morphine and pethidine but without the euphoria caused by these narcotics and may be given parenterally, orally or by suppository.

Pentazocine can cause some respiratory depression which is not antagonized by nalorphine but is reversed by naloxone (see page 185). When given in large parenteral doses, pentazocine causes cardiovascular changes such as a rise in pulmonary arterial pressure which has caused some controversy about its usefulness in acute myocardial infarction.

The evidence at the present time is that pentazocine has a low dependence producing potential and does not require the same stringent control as does morphine. It will produce withdrawal symptoms in those dependent on the opiates.

4. *The morphinans.* Levorphanol is a member of the morphinans and is similar to morphine with a more prolonged action and may also be given by mouth. It has little hypnotic or sedative action.

MILD (ANTIPYRETIC) ANALGESICS

These are known also as the antipyretic analgesics as they lower the body temperature in fever. They act especially on pain arising from skin, muscle, bones and joints by raising the pain threshold rather than by affecting psychic processes of pain appreciation and tolerance does not develop. They are relatively ineffective in traumatic or visceral pain. There are three main groups: the salicylates such as sodium salicylate and acetylsalicylic acid; the aniline (para-amino phenol) derivatives such as phenacetin and paracetamol; and the pyrazolone derivatives such as phenylbutazone.

The Salicylates

These are derivatives of salicylic acid which, itself, is too toxic for analgesic use and is used mainly for its local antispetic and keratolytic action. Salicylic acid was originally obtained from salicin, a glycoside in willow bark (*Salix alba*).

Salicylates are normally given by mouth and are rapidly absorbed from the stomach and the upper part of the small intestine. In the acid region of the stomach, the salicylates, though mainly in the non-ionized form (and hence easily absorbed), are not very soluble. In the alkaline small intestine the salicylates are much less ionized though in a far more soluble form (page 5) and so a considerable part of ingested salicylate will be absorbed here.

Salicylates are mainly excreted as salicylic acid though a considerable proportion is conjugated; some with glycine to give salicyluric acid and some to glucuronides. The clearance of salicylic acid from the plasma depends to a great extent upon the original dose of salicylate; low doses may have a half life of 2–5 hours but with high doses this may become as long as 15–30 hours. Renal clearance of salicylate is greatly increased by making the urine alkaline though there is mutual interreaction between the renal clearances of salicylate, uric acid and penicillin.

Pharmacological actions of the salicylates

Salicylates are effective analgesics in the treatment of headache, muscle pains, joint pains and toothache, though the intensity of pain that can be relieved has a much lower ceiling than with the opiates. The salicylates are most effective in relieving pain due to inflammation but their mode of action is obscure, but is probably peripheral on sensory nerve endings rather than central like the action of morphine. Like other anti-inflammatory drugs they uncouple oxidative phosphorylation, inhibit mucopolysaccharide synthesis and cause redistribution of fluid due to changes in cell permeability. They relieve the pain and joint swellings of rheumatic fever though it is argued if they cure it and prevent the cardiac effects.

Salicylates have many other actions, though the connection between them is not known. They reduce fever, but not normal temperature, probably by acting on the hypothalamic heat-regulating centre and increasing heat loss by peripheral vasodilatation and sweating. They stimulate the respiratory centre directly, increasing respiration in rate and depth. They stimulate the pituitary-adrenal system and also inhibit the action of thyroxine. They increase the urinary excretion of nitrogen and amino acids and have a mild hypoglycaemic action. Hyperglycaemia may occur on occasion perhaps due to adrenaline release. The salicylates are uricosuric, preventing the kidney from reabsorbing uric acid though small doses may have the opposite effect. The salicylates inhibit the formation of prothrombin and act as competitive antagonists to vitamin K. This dicoumarol-like action may cause haemorrhagic phenomena. The relationship between the effects of aspirin and similar drugs on prostaglandin synthesis is discussed on page 94.

Types of salicylates

(a) *Sodium salicylate*. This is analgesic, antipyretic and anti-inflammatory. Its major use is in the treatment of rheumatic fever.

(b) *Acetylsalicylic acid* (*aspirin*). This is the acetyl derivative of salicylic acid. It is well absorbed from the gut to give a maximum plasma concentration in $\frac{1}{2}$–1 hour. It is hydrolysed during absorption to give the free salicylate, though some acetylsalicylic acid as such appears in the plasma.

It is one of the most widely used mild analgesics either alone or in combination with other drugs.

(c) *Aspirin modifications*. There are many modifications of aspirin which attempt to modify or minimize the disadvantages, especially those on the gastrointestinal tract (see below). These preparations include buffered, enteric coated, and other pharmaceutical preparations.

There appears to be no overwhelming evidence that any modified preparation of aspirin is less prone to cause symptoms, which may be minimized by taking the drug after meals, either crushed or in a soluble form.

Salicylate toxicity

Therapeutic doses of salicylates can cause gastric irritation, nausea and vomiting. Gastrointestinal bleeding is common but is usually slight, though frank haematemesis can occur. True allergic reactions range from urticaria to anaphylaxis but are not common though subjects with a history of allergy are more at risk. Salicylates have also been implicated in renal disease (see analgesic nephropathy page 192).

Salicylate overdosage is not uncommon. Moderate overdose causes nausea, vomiting, tinnitus, and deafness. Large doses cause hyperpyrexia, convulsions, coma, dehydration and ketosis. The hyperpyrexia has been explained by salicylate-caused inhibition of many ATP-dependent enzyme systems which deprive the cell of high energy phosphate, and so the energy produced by metabolism is dissipated as heat. Interference with Krebs cycle causes accumulation of keto acids. The respiratory stimulation caused by the salicylates produces hyperpnoea and a respiratory alkalosis. In an attempt to compensate, the kidney secretes an alkaline urine. This results in a metabolic acidosis, which, with the dehydration caused by vomiting and diarrhoea, gives the clinical picture of salicylate overdosage.

The treatment is to maintain the urine volume, keeping it alkaline to facilitate salicylate excretion. Bicarbonate or lactate may be given intravenously to reverse the acidosis with careful monitoring of the electrolyte and acid-base balance. The hyperpyrexia may be reduced by cold sponging. Sodium bicarbonate solution may also be used for gastric lavage and some left in the stomach.

The Aniline Derivatives

1. *Phenacetin* (*acetophenetidin*). Phenacetin is an effective analgesic and antipyretic with an activity similar to that of aspirin but has no anti-inflammatory action and is usually given in combination with other drugs such as aspirin, codeine and caffeine.

It is rapidly metabolized *in vivo* to paracetamol (*N*-acetyl-para-amino-phenol), a metabolite with an active analgesic action. Phenacetin is rapidly absorbed by mouth, giving peak plasma concentrations within 1–2 hours of oral administration and is mainly excreted in the urine as free or conjugated paracetamol.

Phenacetin may cause methaemoglobinaemia and haemolytic anaemia. Its role in the causation of renal papillary necrosis associated with the ingestion of large amounts of phenacetin over a long period is controversial but it is probably safe to assume that prolonged consumption is nephrotoxic.

2. *Paracetamol.* Paracetamol is the major metabolite of both acetanilide and phenacetin. It is an effective analgesic and antipyretic with an activity comparable to that of aspirin but, like phenacetin and other aniline derivatives, has no significant anti-inflammatory action.

It is well absorbed by mouth, reaching peak plasma levels in 45–60 minutes and is rapidly conjugated and excreted via the urine.

Paracetamol is relatively non-toxic when taken in therapeutic doses and has not yet been conclusively linked with causing renal damage. The acute administration of large amounts as in suicidal attempts may cause severe and often fatal liver damage.

Analgesic Nephropathy

Much prominence has been given recently to characteristic changes in the renal papillae said to be associated with the taking of large amounts of various mild analgesics. Classically linked with the ingestion of several grams of phenacetin daily for years, some workers have also incriminated aspirin and paracetamol.

The subject is still highly controversial especially as mixtures of drugs rather than single analgesics are often taken and it may be that these combinations are more prone to cause damage. It would seem unwise for a patient to continue for long periods with the ingestion of any mild analgesic save for compelling therapeutic reasons but occasional use is probably harmless.

The Pyrazolone Derivatives (Amidopyrine-like Drugs)

These drugs such as amidopyrine, phenazone and phenylbutazone have analgesic, antipyretic and anti-inflammatory actions but also have serious side effects. Amidopyrine and phenazone, though having activities comparable to those of the salicylates, are too toxic for everyday use, and amidopyrine is used experimentally to cause agranulocytosis. They occur in some patent and proprietary medicines.

1. *Phenylbutazone.* This drug has powerful anti-inflammatory actions with some analgesic and antipyretic effects. It is rapidly and completely absorbed by mouth though is much protein bound, so metabolism and excretion are slow and cumulation can occur.

It is potentially very toxic and can cause agranulocytosis and other blood dyscrasias, oedema due to sodium retention, and gastrointestinal upsets which include peptic ulcer with haemorrhage and perforation. It may also cause enzyme induction (page 13) and interacts with anti-coagulants to displace them from their blood protein binding sites (see page 163). It is used primarily to treat inflammatory joint disease when less dangerous drugs are ineffective, and has replaced colchicine in the treatment of acute gout.

2. *Oxyphenbutazone.* This is a similar compound and the active metabolite of phenylbutazone.

Various Analgesic and Anti-inflammatory Drugs

There are many drugs of value in the treatment of musculoskeletal diseases such as rheumatoid arthritis or osteoarthrosis.

Aspirin, which is the classical drug used, and phenylbutazone have been discussed elsewhere in this chapter.

1. *Indomethacin.* This is an indoleacetic acid derivative with analgesic, anti-inflammatory and antipyretic actions. It is best avoided as a general purpose analgesic and is used only in rheumatoid arthritis and other musculoskeletal disorders though it is uncertain if it has any major advantage when compared with aspirin. It is also useful in gout.

Indomethacin is rapidly absorbed by mouth and excreted mainly in the urine but may take several weeks to achieve its maximum effect. It may also be given by suppository. Indomethacin is especially likely to cause headache, giddiness, vertigo and gastric upsets.

2. *Mefenamic acid.* This is an anthranilic acid derivative with

analgesic, anti-inflammatory and antipyretic actions and is similar in potency to aspirin. It is liable to cause gastrointestinal upsets, especially diarrhoea.

3. *Flufenamic acid.* This is similar to mefenamic acid.

4. *Benorylate.* This new compound is the paracetamol ester of acetylsalicylic acid and appears to be absorbed as the intact molecule from the gut but is then rapidly hydrolysed in the blood to its component metabolites. It appears to be much less prone to cause gastrointestinal bleeding than aspirin and to be therapeutically effective with twice daily dosage. It may be of value in conditions where long-term salicylate therapy is indicated such as rheumatoid arthritis.

5. *Ibuprofen.* This phenylalkanoic acid derivative is said to have mild analgesic, anti-inflammatory and antipyretic actions. The incidence of side effects is not high but dyspepsia and skin rashes have been reported.

6. *Gold.* Although gold has been used for many years in the treatment of rheumatoid arthritis, it is only comparatively recently that studies have established its effectiveness. It is usually given as sodium aurothiomalate by intramuscular injection in prolonged courses and is especially useful in patients with active, progressive rheumatoid disease. Gold accumulates in the body especially in the kidneys and is excreted via the urine and may be detected there for more than a year after the last dose. Toxic effects are common and include stomatitis, dermatitis and gastrointestinal upsets as well as more serious complications such as kidney and liver damage, bone marrow depression and neuritis.

7. *Antimalarial drugs.* Substances such as chloroquine and hydroxychloroquine which are also antimalarials may be used to treat rheumatoid arthritis. Their action is slow of onset and toxicity is common (page 280) characteristically upon the eye.

8. *Corticosteroids.* The advisability of using corticosteroids in inflammatory disease is controversial but low oral doses of compounds such as prednisolone may be valuable. The side effects and complications of corticosteroid therapy are discussed on page 111.

9. *Immunosuppressive drugs.* Rheumatoid arthritis and other more potentially fatal conditions such as lupus erythematosus may be auto-immune diseases and suppression of the immune response has been used in treatment. This can be achieved by the

corticosteroids or with cytotoxic drugs (page 289 ff), especially cyclophosphamide, azathioprine and methotrexate.

10. D-*penicillamine*. This penicillin derivative enhances copper excretion and is classically used to treat Wilson's disease (hepato-lenticular degeneration). It has recently been reported to be effective in the treatment of rheumatoid arthritis though its mode of action is not known and may be due to chelation of copper, dissociation of macroglobulins, inhibition of collagen synthesis or an antiviral action.

The onset of anti-rheumatoid effect is slow and the incidence of side effects high. These include gastric upset, skin rashes, renal and blood toxicity.

REFERENCES

Beckett, A. H. & Casy, A. F. (1962) The testing and development of analgesic drugs. In *Progress in Medicinal Chemistry*, **2**, 43. Ellis, G. P. & West, G. B. (eds.). London: Butterworth.

Beckett, A. H. & Casy, A. F. (1964) Analgesics and their antagonists: Biochemical aspects and structure-activity relationships. In *Progress in Medicinal Chemistry*, **4**, 171. Ellis, G. P. & West, G. B. (eds.). London: Butterworth.

HYPNOTIC AND SEDATIVE DRUGS

Both hypnotic and sedative drugs depress the central nervous system, but a sedative (Lat. *sedare*, settle) is a drug that soothes whereas a hypnotic is a drug which induces sleep (*Gk. hupnotikos*, producing sleep). Tranquillizers (page 225) relieve anxiety and agitation without any general central nervous depression. The narcotic analgesics (page 181) produce sleep and relieve pain but most other hypnotics have no analgesic action.

It is difficult to decide to which group many drugs belong and some may be used in several capacities depending on the dose and the time of day that they are given.

The precise nature of sleep is ill understood, but the need for it is self evident and hypnotics may help a patient in difficulty. These difficulties are often emotional as well as physical, and elimination of cause is essential in the treatment of insomnia.

The ideal hypnotic. This should reliably produce a natural sleep when taken by mouth or by injection. It should not be dangerous in overdose or produce side effects like residual sedation (hang-over) or drug dependence.

The mode of action of hypnotics. This is discussed more fully with the individual drugs. In their full range of action hypnotics are central nervous depressants closely resembling the volatile anaesthetics but the therapeutic effect corresponds to the first stage of anaesthesia only (page 212). The sensation of pain persists till consciousness is abolished so they are of little use if pain is present.

The Barbiturates

The barbiturates are the most commonly used hypnotics and sedatives. They are derivatives of barbituric acid, a condensation product of malonic acid and urea (malonyl urea). Barbituric acid is not a hypnotic but substitution of various radicals at carbon-5 in the diagram produces the barbiturates which are hypnotic.

	r_1	r_2
Barbitone (Veronal)	O—R—ethyl	ethyl
Phenobarbitone (Luminal)	O—R—ethyl	phenyl
Amylobarbitone (Amytal)	O—R—ethyl	isoamyl
Pentobarbitone (Nembutal)	O—R—ethyl	methylbutyl
Butobarbitone (Soneryl)	O—R—ethyl	butyl
Quinalbarbitone (Seconal)	O—R—allyl	methylbutyl
Thiopentone (Pentothal)	S—R—ethyl	methylbutyl

The chemical structure of the barbiturates.

The longer the side chain at carbon-5, the more lipid-soluble is the barbiturate and the greater the ease with which it will pass the blood–brain barrier to affect the central nervous system, so its potency will be greater though its duration of action will be shorter.

Some barbiturates, such as thiopentone, have a sulphur atom replacing the oxygen atom at carbon-2 in the barbituric acid nucleus which makes them exceptionally lipid soluble and potent.

Barbiturates can produce depression of the central nervous system ranging from mild sedation to full surgical anaesthesia. The precise mode of action is not known but they seem to alter the neurophysiological properties of the sleep mechanism, depressing the activity of the brain so lowering its oxygen consumption and use of high energy phosphates. This results in the raising of the threshold of excitability of the neurone due to stabilization of the cell membrane.

Barbiturates are thought to depress the reticular system. This diffuse network of cells in the medulla, midbrain, hypothalamus and thalamus appears to be concerned in its lower part with sleep and, via the reticular activating system which has collateral fibres from the main sensory tracts, has activating influences on the cortex.

Absorption and fate

The barbiturates are readily absorbed and freely distributed. Their duration of action depends on the rate of absorption, distribution and elimination which varies from one barbiturate to another according to the length of the side chain. They are destroyed especially in the liver microsomal system (page 12) by oxidation of the carbon-5 substituents. Continued administration of barbiturates stimulates development of these microsomal systems (enzyme induction) which also destroy drugs like phenytoin sodium and dicoumarol (page 13).

The speed of metabolism varies from 50% destruction of phenobarbitone in 20 hours to 50% destruction of hexobarbitone in 6 hours.

The duration of action of the barbiturates was classically divided into:

(a) The very short-acting barbiturates such as thiopentone which is given intravenously and has an action lasting a few minutes (page 218).

(b) The short-acting barbiturates such as quinalbarbitone and cyclobarbitone with actions lasting 3–6 hours.

(c) The medium-acting barbiturates such as pentobarbitone, butobarbitone, amylobarbitone with actions lasting 4–8 hours.

(d) The long-acting barbiturates such as phenobarbitone and barbitone with actions lasting 8–16 hours.

This classification is based mainly on animal experiments and the relevance to clinical use in man is dubious. It is likely that with most of the orally administered barbiturates, including phenobarbitone, the duration of action depends on the amount given and not on the chemical structure. In practice the correct dose is found for each individual, taking into account his susceptibility and any concurrent therapy or influences.

The barbiturates have a wide range of uses including the

induction of sleep; the treatment of anxiety states; in general anaesthesia, and as anticonvulsants. They are contraindicated in depression of the respiratory system; liver or kidney damage; a previous history of sensitization, or acute intermittent porphyria (as they may provoke an attack).

Toxic effects of the barbiturates

In hypnotic doses the barbiturates have very little effect on the circulatory, renal, hepatic or gastrointestinal tracts, though larger doses depress the respiratory centre, block autonomic nerves, depress the vasomotor centre and vascular muscle to cause circulatory failure. Hangover is residual sedation and its occurrence is unpredictable and all hypnotic drugs cause it if the dose is large enough. Other toxic effects are skin rashes and sensitivity reactions; the production of confusional states and automatism especially in the elderly. Drug dependence and tolerance may occur, and is discussed on page 238. Alcohol and the barbiturates should not be taken together for the additive effects may produce severe and even fatal depression of the central nervous system.

Treatment of barbiturate overdosage

Barbiturate overdosage is common, either by accident or with suicidal intent. It is generally agreed by most authorities that the use of analeptics (page 221) has no place in the treatment of barbiturate poisoning.

The essentials of modern treatment are:

(a) Support of the respiration by a clear airway and mechanical assistance if necessary.

(b) The prevention or treatment of shock; maintenance of the circulation, renal function; correction of electrolyte imbalance.

(c) Augmented excretion of the drug by forced alkaline diuresis (for phenobarbitone), peritoneal dialysis or haemodialysis.

(d) Gastric lavage if oral ingestion was a short time previously, but this may hasten gastric emptying so simple aspiration may be better.

Miscellaneous Hypnotics

1. *Ethyl alcohol* (*ethanol*). This may be used as a hypnotic, and is discussed on page 205.

2. *Methylpentynol*. This is an alcohol taken in capsules or as an elixir to give a mild sedative and hypnotic action. It is of dubious value.

3. *Paraldehyde*. This is a cyclic ether formed by the polymerization of acetaldehyde. It is an offensive, irritant liquid which crystallizes at 11°C. Paraldehyde may be given orally, intramuscularly or rectally and is a safe hypnotic, not prone to depress the cardiac function or respiration. It produces hypnosis in 15 minutes for 4–8 hours.

Paraldehyde is mainly metabolized by the liver but some 10–30% is excreted via the breath and smells offensively. It is not self sterile and decomposes in storage of 6 months or so to form acetic acid which, if injected, can cause sterile abscesses. It will also dissolve polystyrene so must not be used in disposable syringes.

Paraldehyde is useful as the occasional hypnotic in alcoholism and the convulsions of epilepsy, tetanus or eclampsia.

4. *Chloral hydrate* $C.Cl_3$. $CH(OH)_2$). Chloral hydrate was the first synthetic hypnotic and was made in 1869. It is soluble, colourless, crystalline, hygroscopic and liquifies at 50–58°C.

It is dispensed as a solution and given orally, but has a bitter pungent taste and is a gastric irritant. Chloral hydrate is readily absorbed and acts in 30 minutes for 6–8 hours. It is metabolized in the body to trichlorethanol, which is probably the active substance, and is finally conjugated with glucuronic acid and excreted via the urine as urocholalic acid where it may give a false positive with Fehling's or Benedict's solutions.

5. *Dichloralphenazone*. This is a 2:1 combination of chloral and phenazone. Phenazone is an analgesic and antipyretic but can cause skin eruptions and agranulocytosis.

6. *Triclofos* (*trichloroethyl phosphate*). This is a stable ester of trichloroethanol, the active metabolite of chloral hydrate, and is not unpleasant to take.

7. *Glutethimide*. This is a derivative of glutarimide and has an effective hypnotic action lasting about 6 hours. It can produce nausea and skin rashes and is related to thalidomide.

8. *Tranquillizers* (page 225). Tranquillizers such as meprobamate, nitrazepam, chlordiazepoxide and diazepam also relieve
insomnia but probably by a different mechanism to the barbiturates.

9. *Other hypnotics.* Some drugs are used at times for hypnotic
and sedative effects. These include hyoscine (page 51), the
antihistamines (page 89) and other phenothiazine derivatives
(page 226), the narcotic analgesics (page 181) and bromides
(page 204).

Anticonvulsant Drugs

A convulsion may be defined as a violent involuntary contraction or series of contractions of voluntary muscle. There are many
causes such as epilepsy, tetanus, eclampsia, fever, toxins, hypoglycaemia and anoxia. They are usually due to a transient upset
of cerebral function which is non-recurring after elimination of
the cause. However, the disease may be due to a permanent
cerebral lesion and result in the classical epileptiform pattern.

Epilepsy

This has been recognized as a disease entity since antiquity
when the victim was thought to have been seized by the gods (Gk.
epilepsia, take). The causation was defined by Hughlings Jackson
as a sudden excessive discharge in the grey cells of the brain. The
pattern of the seizure is determined by the localization of the
cerebral abnormality and may vary from subjective phenomena
to the loss of consciousness and convulsions. The classifications of
epilepsy is not clear cut and a textbook of medicine should be
consulted for details, but it may be divided into grand mal, petit
mal, and focal types.

Grand mal is the commonest form of epilepsy and consists of a
typical series of events: the aura, the cry, unconsciousness and a
tonic-clonic fit. Petit mal, which affects mainly children, may be
merely a brief loss of consciousness perhaps with no loss of muscle
tone. Focal epilepsy includes all the other types which are characterized by various localized motor or sensory phenomena. They
include Jacksonian epilepsy and temporal lobe (psychomotor)
epilepsy. Status epilepticus occurs when there is a succession of

fits without the patient recovering between them and will be rapidly fatal if left untreated.

Treatment of epilepsy

Treatment of epilepsy may rarely be specific but if the cause be known, such as a tumour, it may be possible to remove it. Usually it is necessary to use drugs which are not curative but raise the cerebral convulsant threshold. The aim is to establish and maintain a reservoir of drug sufficient to control the convulsions without producing side effects. There is no ideal anticonvulsant drug which would control all convulsion types in an established dosage and produce no untoward side effects. It is necessary to choose one or several drugs and titrate dose-effect in the patient.

Laboratory testing of potential anti-epileptic drugs is very difficult and usually involves a battery of tests. Convulsions in animals may be induced by electrical means, by drugs (e.g. leptazol, strychnine, picrotoxin) or by a variety of other procedures and the capability of a potential anti-epileptic to suppress these seizures is then measured. Most anti-epileptic drugs act in part at least by suppressing activity in neighbouring neurones to an epileptogenic focus and thus blocking the spread of the abnormal electrical discharge, but direct action on the neuronal focus itself may occur with some drugs. Five major groups of anti-convulsant drugs have the chemical structure CO.N.CO.C in common. These are the barbiturates, the hydantoins, the oxazolidines, the phenylacetylureas and the succinimides. Acetazolamide and sulthiame can be considered as derivatives of sulphanilamide. Within each group there is little difference in type of action save in dosage and liability to side effects.

1. *Barbiturates*. These are used mainly for grand mal and may make petit mal worse.

(i) Phenobarbitone: this drug probably acts by stabilizing neuronal membranes and depressing synaptic transmission and is the drug of first choice in grand mal. It has no serious side effects other than sedation which goes if amphetamine is also given. It can cause ataxia, vertigo, blurred vision, allergic rashes, and the occasional sleeplessness.

(ii) Methylphenobarbitone: this drug is probably broken down to phenobarbitone in the liver and has no increased advantages.

(iii) Primidone: the activity of primidone depends in part on its biotransformation to phenobarbitone but as it has an effect on psychomotor epilepsy which phenobarbitone may make worse, it probably has some independent action. Primidone may cause drowsiness, ataxia, vertigo and vomiting as well as a megaloblastic anaemia responsive to folic acid.

2. *Hydantoin derivatives.* These are used in most forms of epilepsy with the exception of petit mal.

(i) Phenytoin: this drug is given mainly orally as phenytoin sodium, though there is a parenteral form. Absorption is slow and maximal plasma concentration does not occur till twelve hours or more after a single dose. Blood levels of more than 10 μg/ml are necessary for an anticonvulsant action and this level may not be reached for 6–10 days. Phenytoin is excreted via the urine, saliva and bile (where some may be reabsorbed).

Toxic effects occur at a blood level of more than 30 μg/ml and include gastric distress, nausea and insomnia especially at the start of treatment. Cerebellar dysfunction may be manifest by nystagmus, diplopia, slurred speech and ataxia, and could be mistaken for alcoholic poisoning. Gum hypertrophy may occur especially in children and hirsutism may be troublesome in young females. More serious side effects are those of hypersensitivity which ranges from a mild rash and transient adenitis similar to German measles, to an exfoliative dermatitis. A megaloblastic anaemia sometimes results especially in the pregnant patient and is reversed by folic acid and may be due to phenytoin acting as a competitive antagonist to folic acid (see also page 146).

(ii) Methoin: this is similar to phenytoin but is said to give no gum hypertrophy but be more likely to cause drowsiness and blood changes.

There are also various fixed dosage forms of hydantoins and barbiturates. Apart from the major disadvantage of inflexibility, the hydantoin level will not remain constant as the enzymes which destroy barbiturates will destroy hydantoins too (see enzyme induction, page 13).

3. *Oxazolidine derivatives (diones).* These may act on the thalamus to raise the threshold for seizure discharge following stimulation as well as having effects on the cortex. They are given orally and include troxidone and the similar paramethadione. They are well absorbed and freely distributed. Metabolism occurs

204 PHARMACOLOGY

in the liver and excretion is via the urine. They are of especial use in petit mal.

Untoward effects include hiccough and nausea, day blindness and photophobia with glaring vision (hemeralopia) in which objects glow and sparkle in the light. More serious effects are exfoliative dermatitis, blood dyscrasias and kidney damage leading to a nephrotic syndrome.

4. *Acetylurea derivatives.* These drugs are effective in psychomotor epilepsy as well as other types. They include such drugs as phenacemide and pheneturide but they are so toxic as not to be drugs of first choice.

5. *Succinimide derivatives.* These drugs such as phensuximide and ethosuximide are very effective in petit mal and psychomotor epilepsy though they can make associated grand mal worse. They can give rise to sleepiness, headache, vomiting, dream states and haematuria.

6. *Carbonic anhydrase inhibitors.* (See also pp. 167, 172.) These sulphonamide derivatives inhibit brain carbonic anhydrase and include acetazolamide and sulthiame. They are of use in grand mal, focal and temporal lobe epilepsy.

7. *Benzodiazepines.* These psychotropic drugs have anticonvulsant properties and are discussed on page 229.

8. *Bromides.* These are historically important but are rarely used these days save in epilepsy that is refractive to other drugs. They are readily absorbed and distributed throughout the whole of the body in the extracellular fluid. Bromide is treated like chloride in the body and the rate of absorption and excretion (which is very slow) depends on the chloride intake. Bromide must replace chloride to a considerable extent to be effective and will depress the whole of the central nervous system, decreasing motor restlessness, causing sedation but not analgesia. Consequently there is no effect till the bromide concentration has built up and single doses are useless. Three grammes of potassium bromide daily will be effective in a week and give toxic signs in a month. These toxic signs or bromism are very insidious and are manifest by depression, irritability, tremors, incoordination, headache, anorexia, foul breath, indigestion, constipation, mucus in the nose, mouth and eyes and also acneiform rashes on the face and trunk. Toxicity appears at blood levels of 100 mg/100 ml (12–15 mEq/l) and is treated by the administration of chloride.

9. *Various drugs.* Many other drugs have been tried in the treatment of epilepsy. These include amphetamine which reduces attacks of petit mal perhaps by decreasing tension; carbamazepine; beclamide; aminoglutethimide; corticotrophin, corticosteroids, and tranquillizers.

In addition to medication, there must be a careful consideration of the patient and his social adjustment. The pattern of the epilepsy must be carefully investigated and treated accordingly. Grand mal and the focal types first be treated with barbiturates and a hydantoin added later if needed. If this is not effective, the succinimides should be tried.

Petit mal is treated with oxazolidines or succinimides as phenobarbitone may make it worse. Tranquillizers or amphetamine may be of help. Psychomotor epilepsy may respond to phenytoin, primidone or phenacemide.

Status epilepticus can be treated with intravenous diazepam as the drug of choice though other drugs can be used such as intramuscular paraldehyde, phenobarbitone sodium, phenytoin sodium or intravenous anaesthetics with mechanical aids to respiration if necessary.

ETHYL ALCOHOL (ETHANOL)

The importance of ethanol is perhaps more social than therapeutic, but it does have useful hypnotic, antiseptic and other actions. Its availability to the lay public as a tranquillizer may be beneficial or the cause of dependence and warrants a good knowledge of its properties.

Alcohol as a beverage. Ethanol forms an important part of many drinks and, in some cases, is the reason for their ingestion. The amount of alcohol in these beverages is often quoted with reference to proof spirit which is taken to be 100° proof and contains 57% of ethanol by volume (50% in the U.S.A.). Whisky, for example, is usually 70° proof (or 30 under proof) which is approximately 40% by volume. Beers contain some 3–15% and wines some 8–15% of ethanol by volume. Fortified wines, such as sherry, contain approximately 20% ethanol. The pharmacology of alcoholic drinks is very complicated and not the same as with simple solutions of ethanol for they contain many other substances such as higher alcohols, ethers and aldehydes which may influence the body response.

Apart from alcoholic drinks, ethanol is available in many different preparations and concentrations and the standard works such as the *British Pharmacopoeia* and the *British Pharmaceutical Codex* should be consulted for details. The sale is complicated by Excise Duty and the precautions taken to avoid non-payment.

Pharmacology of ethanol

Ethanol is a clear liquid which mixes with water to give a rise in temperature and a contraction in volume. It is inflammable in concentrations greater than 50%.

Taken orally, it is rapidly absorbed from the stomach and small intestine but the rate varies greatly and depends on such factors as time since previous food, the fat and carbohydrate content of the stomach and the nature of the beverage itself especially the concentration of ethanol. Ethanol is absorbed fastest on an empty stomach when in moderate concentrations (say 10–15%). Peak blood levels occur $\frac{1}{2}$–2 hours after a single dose.

Ethanol is distributed through the body fluids in proportion to their water content. Small amounts pass unchanged into the urine and alveolar air to form the basis of some medicolegal tests (see below).

Some 90–95% of absorbed ethanol is metabolized in the liver. It is first converted by alcohol dehydrogenase to acetaldehyde which is further converted to acetate (acetylCo-A) by aldehyde dehydrogenase.

The acetate then enters the tricarboxylic acid cycle and is metabolized to CO_2 and H_2O.

The rate of conversion of alcohol to acetaldehyde reaches a maximum when the dehydrogenase system is saturated which occurs with blood levels of about 0·1% alcohol. The maximum rate of conversion for an individual is fairly constant and is approximately 10 ml ethanol/hour.

Main actions of ethanol

(a) *The central nervous system.* Ethanol depresses the central nervous system and, with increasing dose, the subject passes through all the stages of anaesthesia. The higher centres controlling social behaviour and functional patterns are affected first and the release of inhibitions may give the appearance of stimulation. Co-ordination, concentration and skill are soon affected, but later the grosser signs of intoxication, such as stupor and coma, occur. Death results from depression of respiration and the cardiovascular system due to impairment of the medullary centres (Table VII).

TABLE VII. The Behavioural Changes of Acute Alcoholism

Type of Behaviour	Blood Level of Alcohol (mg/100 ml Blood)
—Dead	500
—Dead Drunk	400
—Dazed & Dejected	300
—Dizzy & Delirious	200
—Delighted & Devilish	100
Limit under Road Safety Act 1967	80
—Dry & Decent	

(b) *Other actions of ethanol.* Ethanol has a number of actions on other body systems. It depresses the heat regulatory centre and so diminishes the power of the body to conserve heat. This cooling effect is enhanced by the vasodilatation brought about by ethanol, and hypothermia may result if the environmental conditions are cold. The vasodilatation may cause subjective feelings of warmth and the use of alcoholic drinks to warm a cold person is based on this falsely attributed phenomenon. The use of alcohol as a stimulant in a collapsed person is also falsely based, though concentrated solutions may reflexly accelerate the pulse and respiration by stimulation of the stomach.

Alcoholic drinks may be of use to stimulate psychic secretion of gastric juice via stimulation of the taste buds and the hypnotic effect will lessen any emotional upsets. High concentrations may irritate the gut and so should be avoided in those with peptic ulcer.

Ethanol acts as a diuretic not only by virtue of the fluid bulk with which it is usually ingested but it also inhibits directly vasopressin secretion (page 105).

Ethanol may cause some dilatation of the coronary vessels but not enough to be clinically very useful.

The alleged stimulant effect of ethanol on sexual performance may be due to the abolition of inhibitions but may be summarized as '. . . provokes the desire, but it takes away the performance . . .' (Macbeth II.iii).

Ethanol may also be used as an antiseptic and disinfectant (page 301).

The medicolegal aspects of ethanol

1. *Acute alcoholic poisoning.* This needs no detailed description as most of the effects have been discussed above. Other causes may present a similar picture especially if associated with the previous ingestion of some alcoholic drink. These include carbon monoxide poisoning, overdose of barbiturate, diabetic coma, concussion and head injury, cerebral haemorrhage.

Acute alcoholic poisoning may be diagnosed by both behavioural and chemical tests, though the former have many pitfalls unless the normal performance of the subject is known.

Treatment includes (when necessary) aspiration to empty the stomach, sedation with paraldehyde or chlorpromazine (not barbiturates or opiates) and general nursing care. Claims for other treatment such as intravenous pyridoxine or fructose are suspect.

2. *Chronic alcoholism.* This is a form of drug abuse (page 238)

and the cause of various psychotic states and physical ill health. The mental disturbances range progressively from minor social lapses to florid psychoses. Sudden withdrawal of alcohol is especially likely to precipitate acute psychotic episodes. The physical ill health has many root causes especially if associated with nutritional deficiencies. There may be chronic gastritis, fatty change of the liver and kidneys and a characteristic polyneuropathy.

There is actual tolerance by the central nervous system of the continuously high level of blood alcohol and excretion is not markedly different from that of the abstainer. Other organs such as the gastric mucosa and the liver do not show the same degree of tolerance. There is also an apparent tolerance to the effects of alcohol due to social and behavioural adaptation.

3. *Driving.* It has been shown conclusively that driving skill deteriorates with even the smallest amount of alcohol in the blood. The relevance of this to accidents is obvious and many countries have laid down arbitrary levels of blood alcohol which, if exceeded, make it an offence to be in charge of a motor vehicle.

Under the Road Safety Act 1967 it is an offence to be in charge of a motor vehicle if the blood level of alcohol exceeds 80 mg/100 ml blood.

In the breathalyser test, a measured quantity of breath passes through a glass tube containing particles of silica coated with potassium dichromate and sulphuric acid. In the presence of alcohol, the yellow dichromate changes to green chromic sulphate. If the green change extends far enough up the tube, this indicates a blood level of more than 80 mg alcohol/100 ml blood and is *prima facie* evidence for further investigations which, if corroborative, lead to prosecution under the Act.

Disulfiram (tetraethylthiuram disulphide). This drug blocks the action of aldehyde dehydrogenase which converts acetaldehyde to acetate.

By itself it is relatively non-toxic but, if ethanol be taken, disulfiram prevents further oxidation of acetaldehyde produced by the metabolic degradation of ethanol. This rise in blood acetaldehyde causes flushing, palpitations, giddiness and nausea.

Disulfiram has found some use in preventing an alcoholic from taking spirits or other drinks containing ethanol for fear of the result.

Metronidazole (see page 283) also inhibits aldehyde dehydrogenase, and may produce alcohol intolerance.

Methyl alcohol (*methanol*). Methanol is the chief toxic constituent of methylated and surgical spirits and is an important cause of poisoning.

Methanol is very slowly oxidized to give formaldehyde and formates which accumulate and are very toxic. The onset of symptoms is slow and may take 12–24 hours when lassitude, nausea and vomiting occur followed by confusion, coma and death. There may also be visual disturbances leading to optic atrophy and blindness.

Due to the accumulation of acid metabolites, there is a marked acidosis and a greatly decreased alkali reserve. Poisoning is best treated by intravenous bicarbonate or lactate to reverse the acidosis. The giving of ethanol (sufficient to get a blood concentration of 100 mg/100 ml) will help as this is metabolized by the same pathways and prevents the conversion of methanol to formates by substrate competition.

REFERENCES

Oswald, I. (1968) Drugs and sleep. *Pharmacological Reviews*, **20**, 273.

Spinks, A. & Waring, W. S. (1963) Anticonvulsant drugs. In *Progress in Medicinal Chemistry*, **3**, 261. Ellis, G. P. & West, G. B. (eds.). London: Butterworth.

GENERAL ANAESTHETICS

A general anaesthetic is an agent used to produce a reversible loss of consciousness and sensation. Surgical anaesthesia may be defined as the total unawareness of environment without appreciation of pain or other sensory perception and without memory of the experience.

Drugs have been used since the earliest times to relieve the pain of operative procedures but not until the middle of the last century was there any satisfactory method. The use of ether in 1842 by Crawford Long and by Morton in 1846, and the use of nitrous oxide by Horace Wells in 1844 gave rise to much controversy. Anaesthesia developed rapidly, however, especially with the use of chloroform in 1847 by Simpson and by John Snow for Queen Victoria at the birth of Prince Leopold ('chloroform a la reine').

The mode of action of general anaesthetics

This is a very disputed and unsettled subject but the fundamental action appears to be a reversible and partly non-specific depression of cell function. It is interesting to note that inert gases such as helium, krypton, xenon and nitrogen, at certain pressures, display the typical properties of anaesthetic gases. This may be of importance in deep sea diving as, at 5 atmospheres of nitrogen (45 metres of water), signs of central nervous impairment can occur. Helium–oxygen mixtures are better in this respect as they have less depressant action than nitrogen–oxygen mixtures.

212   PHARMACOLOGY

Most theories of general anaesthesia are now only of historical interest though that proposed by Overton and Meyer (1899–1901) still explains many of the observed facts. They correlated the narcotic potency with fat solubility and showed that, the greater the solubility in fat, the greater the narcotic power. Although many homologous aliphatic series have graded narcotic powers, some narcotics are not fat soluble and some fat-soluble compounds are not narcotics. The classical Overton-Meyer theory has been modified by more recent theories such as that of Ferguson who related the thermodynamic potential of the anaesthetic (the percentage saturation of a tissue phase) with its potency.

On some tissues, general anaesthetics affect conduction, depress transmitter release, block autonomic ganglia and reduce the sensitivity of the motor end plate. They depress enzyme systems but the concentrations needed are high and although oxygen consumption falls, this could be secondary to reduced neuronal activity rather than a primary cause.

Some theories stress interference with cell membranes. The pores in the cell membranes might be blocked by the drug thus preventing the passage of ions across it. One intriguing theory is that of Miller and Pauling who say that the anaesthetic forms microcrystals of ice (clathrates) which interfere with synaptic transmission and the excitability of neuronal membranes. These crystals are stabilized at body temperatures by charged side chains of proteins.

It is obvious that no one theory of anaesthesia is satisfactory but neither are they necessarily mutually exclusive and perhaps further evidence will lead to unification.

The stages of anaesthesia

All anaesthetics produce basically the same effect on the central nervous system and their selective action on the higher centres is probably not due to any greater concentration but to a greater susceptibility. As administration continues, there is a progressive and irregularly descending paralysis starting at the cortex, basal ganglia and cerebellum; then the spinal cord (first the sensory and then the motor tracts from below upwards) and finally the medulla. This is a phylogenetic scale with the most recently developed and complex functions being affected first. It results clinically in four stages of anaesthesia being recognized according to the degree of paralysis, and which are best understood when related to the phylogenetic scale mentioned above. They are correlated to various physical signs and were originally described for ether anaesthesia unmodified by other drugs. The modern practice of multiple drug anaesthesia greatly affects the original classical signs and the use of muscle relaxants completely alters the significance of changes in muscle tone.

Stage One (of analgesia). The patient is conscious and can talk and obey commands. There is only partial analgesia.

Stage Two (of delirium or excitement). This is characterized by unconsciousness and inhibition of the higher centres. Reflexes are still present and may be exaggerated. Violent muscular reactions can occur if this stage is not expertly managed.

Stage Three (of surgical anaesthesia). This is divided into four planes and the required depth depends on the particular operation. The planes are characterized by changes in respiration, eye movement and muscle tone.

Stage Four (of medullary paralysis). This is a terminal event and death rapidly follows by failure of circulation and respiration.

The recovery of the patient occurs in roughly the reverse order and the first clear signs are usually dilatation of the pupil and the return of the conjunctival reflex followed by the coughing and vomiting reflexes.

Methods of administration of an anaesthetic

This is a highly skilled and complex task and no details are given here. Anaesthesia may be produced by the inhalation of a volatile or gaseous compound; by intravenous injection; or more rarely by rectal administration. Inhalation anaesthetics are either liquid at room temperature and pressure and have to be volatilized for administration or are those which are gases at normal room temperature and pressure and so are dispensed under pressure in cylinders.

The ideal anaesthetic

Clinical anaesthetic practice has three objects: to provide hypnosis, analgesia and muscle relaxation. To achieve this the administration of an anaesthetic falls into three phases: the induction of anaesthesia to bring the patient to the correct level for operation (see also Premedication, page 220); the maintenance of anaesthesia during the operation; and, finally, the recovery from anaesthesia.

As with so many drugs it is profitable to consider what properties are desirable in an anaesthetic and to bear these in mind when considering the individual drugs. The ideal anaesthetic must provide the hypnosis, analgesia and muscular relaxation necessary for an operation and may be considered under the following headings:

(i) *The patient*. He needs a fast, pleasant induction by a non-irritant gas with no unpleasant smell. He wants a comfortable recovery but above all, he wants a safe anaesthetic.

(ii) *The surgeon*. He wants a non-explosive gas in case diathermy is used (as well as the obvious safety reasons). Capillary bleeding should not increase and muscle relaxation must be adequate.

(iii) *The anaesthetist*. He wants a drug with a wide safety margin with minimal upset of normal physiology yet potent enough to allow adequate oxygen to be given. It should be rapidly absorbed and excreted to facilitate control of body concentration and so is most likely to be given by inhalation.

(iv) *The manufacturer*. He wants a cheap, easily made drug, unaffected by storage and patentable by him.

No ideal anaesthetic has yet been found and the nearest approach is a combination of drugs in such a way that the maximum advantages are gained. The requirements of sleep, analgesia and muscular relaxation are often obtained with separate drugs.

Uptake and distribution of the inhalational anaesthetics

As the whole of the blood passes through the lungs every thirty seconds, the uptake of inhaled anaesthetic is very rapid and is second in speed to intravenous administration. The concentration of anaesthetic in the pulmonary arterial bed will approximate to that of the alveolar air, but as the anaesthetic is at first rapidly taken up by the tissues, the initial venous concentration will be low. As the tissues become saturated and so take up less anaesthetic, the venous concentration rises and so the amount taken up in the lungs falls.

The actual amount taken up also depends on the solubility of the gas in blood. The very soluble gases are so rapidly and completely taken up (i.e. before full equilibration) that the alveolar concentration (and so the diffusion gradient across the pulmonary capillary bed) cannot build up with successive breaths and the theoretical possible blood concentration is not reached for a long time. As the level of anaesthesia depends on the amount in the brain and this in turn depends on the tension gradient in the blood, anaesthetics like ether which are very soluble tend to take a long time to enter the brain and induction of anaesthesia is slow. Anaesthesia may be hastened by increasing the concentration of drug inhaled but this is limited by the irritation caused by some anaesthetics and the need to avoid anoxia. With the less soluble anaesthetics such as nitrous oxide, the blood is quickly saturated and the blood concentration rises to the expected values and so brain concentration increases rapidly and induction of anaesthesia is quicker.

The amount of anaesthetic taken up by a particular tissue also depends on the blood supply which in the brain is very high and is comparable to that of the heart and far in excess of that of muscle.

When administration of anaesthetic stops, elimination occurs in the reverse order and is quickest from organs with a good blood supply.

The individual anaesthetic agents

1. *Diethyl ether (anaesthetic ether)* $(C_2H_5)_2.O$. Ether is a very volatile colourless liquid (b.p. 35°C) giving off an irritant, inflammable and explosive vapour which, as it is heavy, sinks to the floor where low level sources of ignition may be important. Ether decomposes on storage especially when exposed to light and air and the presence of decomposition products, aldehydes and peroxides, make it even more likely to explode.

Ether is simple to give by the open, partial or complete rebreathing methods though its volatility can be troublesome in hot climates. As ether is so soluble in body fluids, a large amount has to be taken up for anaesthesia so induction is slow and is normally achieved by the use of thiopentone. Ether is distributed throughout the body, is not metabolized, and is eliminated mainly via the expired air.

Ether is very irritant to the respiratory tract and much mucus and secretions are formed though are considerably lessened by preoperative atropinization. The irritation of the respiratory tract may initially cause laryngospasm. Ether is a potent anaesthetic and can depress the patient through all the stages of anaesthesia even when combined with sufficient oxygen to avoid anoxia. The heart rate, blood pressure, and blood sugar may rise during the use of ether owing to vigorous sympathoadrenal discharge. There is also marked peripheral vasodilation. As the circulatory system remains relatively unimpaired even when enough anaesthetic is given to stop respiration, ether is said to be a safe anaesthetic. Adrenaline and noradrenaline may be given safely during ether anaesthesia. Ether also has a relaxant effect on muscle synergistic with tubocurarine which can be of clinical significance.

2. *Chloroform CHCl₃*. Although chloroform is seldom used nowadays, it may (with other old-fashioned anaesthetics and practices) still find a place in some isolated parts. It is a clear, volatile liquid, boiling at 61°C. It is non-explosive though the vapour, if exposed to a flame, decomposes to phosgene. It is unstable in storage. Chloroform is very potent with a short induction period and a long recovery period, and may be administered by the open or closed methods with full surgical anaesthesia obtained in 2–3 minutes.

Chloroform is irritant to the respiratory tract but, as smaller concentrations are used than with ether, this is not so much a problem. The blood pressure gradually and continuously falls during chloroform anaesthesia due to depression of the vasomotor centre and myocardium. Chloroform is also likely to cause ventricular fibrillation early in the anaesthesia due to sensitization of the heart to endogenous or injected adrenaline. Chloroform can also cause respiratory arrest but, in contrast to ether, this is associated with circulatory depression.

Chloroform has several major toxic effects on the liver: repeated small doses cause cirrhosis; used in anaesthesia it can cause fatty degeneration of the liver, heart and kidneys and the safe time limit for the duration of anaesthesia is about 45–60 minutes. In the so-called delayed chloroform poisoning which occurs on the 1st to 3rd day after operation, there is liver failure due to central necrosis.

3. *Halothane CHBrCl.CF₃*. Halothane is a clear odourless fluid which is stable, volatile (b.p. 50°C), non-inflammable and

non-explosive (under normal conditions). It is extremely potent and needs special apparatus to control the inhaled concentration, and a 2–4% concentration induces anaesthesia which can be maintained by a ½–1½% concentration. Induction is smooth and there is no increase in salivary or bronchial secretions. Like ether it is preferentially soluble in fat. Recovery is fairly rapid, halothane being exhaled unchanged and the incidence of post-operative nausea and vomiting is low.

Halothane can cause hypotension due to ganglion blockade, increase in vagal tone and direct depression of the myocardium. It may also cause arrhythmias and sensitize the myocardium to adrenaline. Halothane is synergistic with the relaxant effect of tubocurarine. Its great potency makes it dangerous in unskilled hands though its overall record of safety is superior to most anaesthetics. It is also expensive and used in closed circuit anaesthesia.

Although similar to chloroform there is no unequivocal evidence of liver damage being caused, though it may cause very rarely a sensitivity type of hepatic reaction, especially on repeated administration, which is virtually indistinguishable from acute virus hepatitis.

4. *Methoxyflurane* $CH_3.O.CF_2.CHCl_2$. This halogenated anaesthetic is a clear colourless liquid with a boiling point of 104·7°C. It is non-inflammable, non-explosive and stable in the presence of soda lime. It has a low volatility hence induction is slow and recovery is also prolonged. It is a very potent anaesthetic, non-irritant, and produces good muscular relaxation. It consistently produces a fall in blood pressure proportional to the dose given. It is a strong analgesic in subanaesthetic doses.

5. *Trichloroethylene.* Trichloroethylene is a colourless liquid with a b.p. of 87°C but in anaesthetic practice is coloured blue to distinguish it from chloroform. It is non-inflammable, non-explosive and non-irritant. It is likely to cause breathing irregularities and severe cardiac arrhythmias and must not be used in a closed circuit with soda lime (which is used to absorb CO_2) as it will then decompose to produce neurotoxic compounds. The use of trichloroethylene is waning but it is still used as a self-administered analgesic in midwifery and as a supplement to nitrous oxide.

6. *Ethyl chloride* $CH_3.CH_2.Cl$. Ethyl chloride has a b.p. of 12·5°C and is kept under pressure in a special glass bottle with a

spring-loaded nozzle. It is inflammable and extremely potent with a very small safety margin. It is used mainly to induce general anaesthesia but may also be used as a local analgesic. When sprayed on the skin, the ensuing evaporation causes cooling to produce a localized analgesia which is neither marked nor long lasting.

7. *Nitrous oxide N_2O.* Nitrous oxide is a colourless gas with a faint sweetish smell and is dispensed in liquid form under 45 atmospheres of pressure in royal-blue steel cylinders. It is non-explosive and non-inflammable but will support combustion as high temperatures cause it to dissociate into nitrogen and oxygen (though this dissociation does not occur in the body). It is rapidly absorbed and excreted via the lungs, though a small amount is excreted via the skin.

The mechanism of action of nitrous oxide is disputed. It was thought to act by purely asphyxial processes but as a mixture of 80% with 20% oxygen causes unconsciousness and analgesia though not full surgical anaesthesia, other mechanisms must be involved also. To get full anaesthesia with nitrous oxide alone, it is necessary to give a higher concentration than 80%, perhaps up to 100%, but this will cause anoxia with cerebral damage if continued for more than 2–3 minutes and many would condemn outright the use of nitrous oxide in this way.

The deeper planes of anaesthesia are more safely reached by nitrous oxide and adequate oxygen with the use of additional agents such as ether, thiopentone, pethidine and muscle relaxants. Nitrous oxide is non-irritating and has no untoward side effects and, if it were not such a weak anaesthetic, would qualify for the title of the Ideal Anaesthetic. The real danger of nitrous oxide is in the production of anoxia and not in the gas itself.

8. *Cyclopropane.* Cyclopropane is a heavy colourless gas with a characteristic ether-like odour. It is dispensed in orange-coloured cylinders as a liquid under pressure. It is inflammable, explosive and used in closed circuit. It is exceptionally potent and induction is rapid, to give an uncomplicated smooth anaesthesia though cardiac irregularities may occur.

9. *Thiopentone sodium* (see also page 197). Thiopentone sodium, structurally, is pentobarbitone with a sulphur atom replacing the oxygen. It is given intravenously, usually to induce anaesthesia, which is then maintained by other agents such as nitrous oxide,

halothane, etc. It may be used as the sole anaesthetic in very short operations such as manipulations or the setting of fractures, but this can be dangerous owing to the possibility of respiratory arrest.

Thiopentone is given as a $2\frac{1}{2}\%$ solution and the dose determined for each patient. When given intravenously thiopentone is quickly taken up by the brain in high concentrations. The effect of an initial dose of 0·25 g lasts only about 10–20 minutes and this comparatively rapid recovery is because thiopentone moves out of the brain to become redistributed in the viscera, body tissues and body fat where it is therapeutically inactive.

Thiopentone is metabolized slowly by the liver and other tissues at the rate of 10–15%/hour. The increasing response to rapid successive doses of thiopentone is due to the filling of the tissue depots so the blood concentration and hence the brain concentration remains high.

Thiopentone Injection B.P. is very irritant and extravenous administration must be avoided. Subcutaneous injection may cause sloughing whilst, if given perineurally (the median nerve is the most common), paralysis will result. Intra-arterial injection causes thrombosis, perhaps with consequent gangrene. Though usually given intravenously, thiopentone may also be administered by rectum.

10. *Propanidid*. This phenoxy-acetic acid derivative (i.e. non barbiturate) is given intravenously as an oily solution and produces anaesthesia of not more than 4–5 minutes and is much used in minor dental and surgical operations.

11. *Methohexitone*. This drug may also be given intravenously either for the induction of general anaesthesia or for short lasting anaesthesia. The rapid recovery makes it suitable for outpatient use.

12. *Ketamine*. This drug is related to the hallucinogen phencyclidine. It produces a state of dissociation from the environment with analgesia, amnesia and light sleep ('dissociative anaesthesia'). Muscle relaxation is poor and the blood pressure and heart rate may rise. Ketamine is said not to depress the laryngeal and pharyngeal reflexes but this is disputed. Ketamine given intravenously produces anaesthesia within a minute to last for 5–10 minutes. Intramuscular administration produces a slower onset of action. Recovery is often slow and may be associated with unpleasant

dreams. Ketamine may be used in diagnostic or short term operations, for induction or as a supplement to other forms of anaesthesia.

Neuroleptanalgesia

If a powerful analgesic such as phenoperidine (page 187) or fentanyl (page 187) is given in combination with droperidol, a neuroleptic drug of the butyrophenone series (page 228), the state of mental indifference and analgesia resulting is known as neuroleptanalgesia. The combination of drugs, given intravenously, allows surgical procedures such as neurological investigations to be carried out with the cooperation of the patient, maintenance of cardiovascular stability and the vital reflexes together with good analgesia and some amnesia for the event though marked respiratory depression may occur. The combination may also be given with light anaesthesia (e.g. nitrous oxide and oxygen) to provide neuroleptanaesthesia.

Premedication

This term embraces the giving of drugs prior to the induction of anaesthesia with three main objects: sedation and amnesia; analgesia; and inhibition of the parasympathetic nervous system. They may be considered under the following two headings:

(i) *Drugs used to cause sedation and analgesia.* These are used for humanitarian reasons as well as to avoid excitement and to give freedom from pain during the initial phases of the anaesthetic. Their effect may last throughout the anaesthesia proper and reduce the amount of anaesthetic necessary. Morphine is commonly used, though some prefer papaveretum which is a total extract of opium alkaloids. Pethidine may be given preoperatively and as an adjuvant to anaesthetic agents such as nitrous oxide. Other drugs used include the barbiturates and tranquillizers such as diazepam.

(ii) *Drugs used to inhibit the parasympathetic system.* These lessen the massive secretions occurring with drugs such as ether and also prevent reflex vagal inhibitory action on the heart. Atropine sulphate is the drug of choice in the elderly and the young, though in others, hyoscine may be used as this give some sedation and anti-emetic effects as well.

It is also important to remember that previously given drugs or disease states may modify the usual response to the anaesthetic agents.

CENTRAL NERVOUS SYSTEM STIMULANTS

Many drugs stimulate the central nervous system but are usually non-specific in their actions and stimulate all levels. There are exceptions such as apomorphine, which stimulates only the vomiting and vasomotor centres. Some drugs such as the monoamine oxidase inhibitors, the tricyclic antidepressants, and amphetamine are used in the treatment of psychological depression and are discussed on page 232.

Analeptics (GK. *ana*, again; *lepticos*, to restore)

An analeptic drug is intended to produce arousal, to improve the rate and depth of breathing, to produce a rise of blood pressure, and a return of depressed reflexes. They are usually non-specific and the respiratory stimulant dose is usually near that causing convulsions. Save for aminophylline (page 223), the analeptics have little place in modern medicine.

Analeptics have been commonly used to stimulate depressed respiration by increasing the depth and rate of breathing and may act directly on the respiratory centre or sensitize it to a rise in P_{CO_2}. They may also stimulate the carotid body receptors. They should not be used in the treatment of respiratory depression due to drugs, though may be of some value in carbon dioxide narcosis of the chronic bronchitis or in respiratory failure of the newborn. They are commonly given intravenously.

1. *Strychnine.* This is alkaloid obtained from the seeds of the tree, *Strychnos nux vomica*. It has no important therapeutic value but has proved a useful research tool into the mode of action of convulsant drugs.

2. *Picrotoxin.* This substance is obtained from the berries of an East Indian plant. The therapeutic ratio is low and there is little appreciable effect till nearly convulsive doses. It has been used in the treatment of barbiturate poisoning though the effect is transient and frequent doses are necessary.

3. *Nikethamide.* This drug is a synthetic derivative of nicotinic

acid and has weak analeptic properties though will cause convulsions if given in large doses. It stimulates all levels of the central nervous system, especially the medulla, and increases respiration in doses that have little other effect. It sensitizes the respiratory centre to carbon dioxide and may also stimulate the carotid body receptors. It has inconsistent effects on the circulation and may cause vasoconstriction and a rise in blood pressure.

Nikethamide is usually given intravenously but sometimes orally. It is used in central nervous depression to stimulate the breathing of chronic bronchitis, or to stimulate respiration in the newborn.

4. *Ethamivan*. The drug is the diethylamide of vanillic acid and is related to nikethamide. It is used as a respiratory stimulant and is preferable to nikethamide.

6. *Lobeline*. This drug is an alkaloid from Lobelia (Indian tobacco) and has general actions like nicotine, (page 54) though much less potent. It stimulates the central nervous system and increases respiration via the carotid sinus mechanism. It has been used in attempts to cure the tobacco habit.

7. *Doxapram*. Doxapram has a direct stimulant action on the respiratory centre and has mild pressor actions due to vasoconstriction. It is one of the drugs of choice if a respiratory stimulant is wanted.

The xanthine derivatives

These are a group of methylated xanthines of which the best known are caffeine, theobromine, and theophylline. They have many properties in common though not all to the same degree. Thy stimulate the central nervous system, have a weak diuretic action, stimulate the myocardium, and relax smooth muscle. These xanthines occur in various plants throughout the world and man has made beverages from them since the earliest times. Caffeine occurs especially in tea and coffee, and theobromine occurs in cocoa.

(i) *Caffeine*. This is the most potent central stimulant of the xanthines and acts especially on the cortex. It reduces reaction time and counteracts fatigue though its effect on learning are negligible. These actions are caused by the amount in several cups of coffee (100–250 mg). Caffeine is also a potent respiratory stimulant. Toxic doses can cause sleeplessness, hallucinations, and even tetanic convulsions.

(ii) *Aminophylline*. Theophylline is less potent as a central stimulant than caffeine but is more powerful as a smooth muscle relaxant, diuretic, and stimulant of the myocardium. It is somewhat insoluble in water but, in combination with ethylenediamine, its solubility and potency are greatly increased (Aminophylline Injection B.P.). It may also be given by suppository.

Aminophylline is not only a fairly potent stimulant to respiration but also causes considerable relaxation of smooth muscle and so can cause pulmonary vasodilatation. It has more diuretic action than the other xanthines and acts partly by reducing the tubular reabsorption of sodium and partly by increasing renal blood flow. This combination of effects makes aminophylline of great use in acute cardiac asthma when it is commonly given intravenously.

REFERENCES

Wylie, W. D. & Churchill Davidson, H. C. (1972). *A Practice of Anaesthesia*, 3rd edn. London: Lloyd Luke.

PSYCHOTROPIC DRUGS

Psychotropic drugs are drugs that act on psychic function, behaviour, or experience. They play an important part in the treatment (and causation) of many mental disorders. They usually provide symptomatic relief only and do not affect disease processes but may so modify the emotional state of the patient as to make him more receptive of other psychological procedures.

The determination of the therapeutic efficiency of drugs used in mental disorder is perhaps more difficult than in any comparable field. In most cases the cause of the human disorder is not known and there is usually no exact animal parallel. Even the classification of the various disorders is controversial and it is not easy to be unequivocal in the diagnosis of the type and severity of the disease process present.

Recent work in the biochemistry of the central nervous system in abnormal mental behaviour may prove to be a more useful approach especially if a characteristic abnormality can be firmly correlated with a particular mental state. There is increasing recognition of inherited or other biochemical defects which can cause central nervous damage which may be prevented by dietary or other means. These include kernicterus, phenylketonuria, hepatolenticular degeneration, congenital porphyria and Vitamin B deficiency neuropathy. A fairly consistent relationship has been observed between the effects of some psychotropic drugs and their action on amine metabolism. However, the hypothesis, for example, that depression occurs when the levels of amines in the brain are reduced and that antidepressant drugs increase these levels is undoubtedly too simple and the final picture is more complex. Certain nervous pathways are being identified with specific modes of behaviour and these pathways may rely upon different amines as neurotransmitters. The balance between transmitter availability and receptor sensitivity determines functional status and as one or more of the amine mediated systems can be involved in various degrees, the resulting picture can be quite complex. A drug, metabolic or pathological influence on these types of pathways, while causing observable and perhaps characteristic behaviour patterns, may not cause sufficient neuropharmacological disturbance to be easily identified in any gross fashion.

It is possible to approach the study of drugs used in the treatment of mental disorder in several ways; each of which has its particular merits. The drugs may be classified according to their chemical structure, their biochemical actions or their predominant clinical use. The last classification will be used here, though more than a brief mention of the types of mental disorder would be out of place. These psychotropic drugs are commonly divided into the tranquillisers and the antidepressants though there is an important third group, the psychodysleptics.

TRANQUILLIZERS

The term tranquillizer is a generic one and is given to a vast variety of drugs of very different types. They reduce agitation and anxiety without producing the hypnosis and clouding of consciousness typical of barbiturates or alcohol and, even if large doses of tranquillizer are given, the patient can still be aroused.

It is difficult to be dogmatic about the types of illness treated with tranquillizers but, in general, the more potent drugs (neuroleptics, major tranquillizers), such as the phenothiazine derivatives, are used for psychotic states. The less potent tranquillizers (anxiolytic sedatives, minor tranquillizers), such as meprobamate and the benzodiazepine derivatives, are used in anxiety and neurotic states. Other drugs such as the barbiturates also play a major role (page 197).

The phenothiazine derivatives

The phenothiazine ring consists of two benzene rings linked by sulphur and nitrogen (see diagram below). Substitutions are usually made at positions 2 and 10 to form a whole range of derivatives of which promethazine was the first. Promethazine was found to be antihistaminic (page 89) and very sedative.

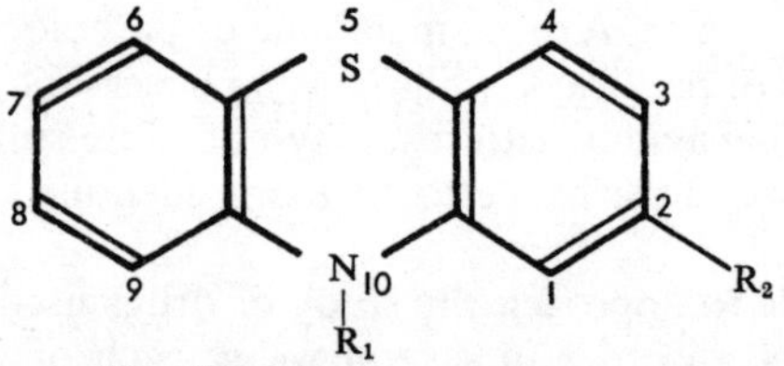

The phenothiazine nucleus

1. *Chlorpromazine.* This is the prototype of the major tranquillizers. It has a $(CH_2)_3.N.(CH_3)_1$ group at R_2 and a Cl group at R_2.

Chlorpromazine is well absorbed by mouth and is rapidly distributed. It is mainly metabolized by hydroxylation or by conjugation with glucuronic acid. Other routes are by the formation of sulphoxides and by demethylation.

Chlorpromazine has a large number of actions whose mechanism is very obscure. It produces marked sedation at first though the patient rapidly becomes tolerant to this There is psychomotor slowing, emotional quieting and affective indifference (the neuroleptic syndrome). Chlorpromazine reduces the response to conditioned stimuli in doses which do not affect the response to unconditioned stimuli, unlike the barbiturates which reduce the response to both kinds of stimuli simultaneously.

Chlorpromazine depresses centres in the hypothalamus and the brain stem though its action on the reticular system is disputed, but is probably to block the connections between the sensory pathways and the reticular formation. Chlorpromazine blocks the action of dopamine at the dopaminergic receptor and so will affect the basal ganglia. Whilst small doses may reduce Parkinsonian tremor, large doses may actually cause it. Chlorpromazine acts as an anti-emetic and antagonizes the stimulation of the chemoreceptor trigger zone by drugs such as morphine. Unlike reserpine, it does not reduce the amounts of 5-HT and noradrenaline in the brain.

Chlorpromazine has strong α-adrenergic and weaker cholinergic blocking properties. It also causes slight ganglion block and is antagonistic to histamine and 5-HT.

Chlorpromazine has a complex action on the cardiovascular system. Hypotension occurs due to inhibition of central nervous responses, peripheral α-adrenergic block causing vasodilatation, and a direct depressant action on the heart. There is also a tachycardia due to the decrease in peripheral resistance and to the atropine-like effects.

Chlorpromazine is a potent local anaesthetic, though is not used for this, and also has quinidine-like actions. It causes relaxation of skeletal muscle and may be useful in spastic conditions. It also causes some pituitary inhibition and hence a variety of endocrine effects.

Although its pharmacological effects last about 8 hours, the effect on behaviour may not be apparent for some weeks and persist for two weeks after cessation of therapy. Phenothiazine derivatives are detectable in the urine for 6–12 months after stopping treatment.

2. *Other phenothiazines.* There are a great variety of phenothiazine derivatives, and depending on the structure of the side chain at R_1, they may be classified in three groups. None is a major advance on chlorpromazine.

(i) Propylamine group: promazine, chlorpromazine, acepromazine, methotrimeprazine, fluopromazine.

(ii) Piperazine group: prochlorperazine, trifluoperazine, fluphenazine, perphenazine.

(iii) Piperidine group: pecazine, thioridazine.

Toxic effects of the phenothiazines. The phenothiazines as a group have a high therapeutic ratio and do not give rise to drug dependence. They may produce drowsiness, lethargy, postural hypotension and extrapyramidal effects such as Parkinsonism, dyskinesia and akathisia. There may be marked lowering of the body temperature due to peripheral vasodilatation and depression of the hypothalamus.

Various blood dyscrasias and dermatological reactions may also occur. An obstructive type of jaundice can result due to damage of the bile canaliculi. This may be a hypersensitivity reaction. The phenothiazines also potentiate many other drugs such as barbiturates, morphine, pethidine, and may cause dangerous interactions.

Uses of the phenothiazines. The phenothiazines are useful in hyperactive and manic states, in schizophrenia, in behavioural disorders, in alcoholism, drug dependence, and as anti-emetics (page 248). They also aid the production of hypothermic states and potentiate the actions of analgesics. They are usually given by mouth though may be given by injection or suppository.

The rauwolfia alkaloids

Rauwolfia alkaloids have long been used in India for their calming and sedative action. Reserpine, an extract of *Rauwolfia serpentina*, is characteristic of the group.

It is readily absorbed by mouth, though its effects are slow in onset and may persist for a long time after the drug is discontinued ('hit-and-run' drug). Reserpine releases tissue amines such as adrenaline, noradrenaline, dopamine, 5-HT and histamine from their storage sites, which may be the explanation of its action on the central nervous system, though the phenothiazines do not have this depleting action.

Reserpine has a calming effect, reducing aggressiveness and producing indifference to the surroundings. It also has some extrapyramidal effects similar to Parkinsonism. Its action on the adrenergic neurone is discussed on page 68.

Reserpine is used especially in the treatment of hypertension (page 149) and psychoneuroses. It has the serious side effect of producing severe mental depression which has led to suicide and some clinicians feel that it should not be used.

Butyrophenones

These compounds such as haloperidol and droperidol are similar in many of their effects to the phenothiazines and may act by mimicking the putative neurotransmitter gamma aminobutyric acid and perhaps by blocking the central actions of the cate-cholamines. Extrapyramidal signs due to block of dopaminergic receptors are frequent but peripheral α-adrenergic block is seen only with high doses and anti-cholinergic effects are slight.

The butyrophenones have similar therapeutic indications as for the phenothiazines (see also 'neuroleptanalgesia' page 220).

Lithium

Lithium salts have recently been shown to be effective in the treatment of manic disorders. Lithium ions are readily absorbed orally and are excreted mainly via the kidney. Lithium can substitute for sodium in the extracellular fluid but as it is not removed from cells by the sodium pump, conduction in excitable tissues will be severely impaired.

The central effects of lithium are not marked in therapeutic doses save in manic patients when the plasma level should be kept at 0·8–1·2 mEq/litre. Although the precise mode of action is not known, lithium appears to decrease the central levels of noradrenaline.

Meprobamate

Meprobamate is a simple aliphatic compound derived from mephenesin. It is readily absorbed and has an action similar to that of the barbiturates and is claimed to depress selectively the limbic system and the thalamus. It is anticonvulsant, reduces the tone of skeletal muscle, and does not affect the autonomic nervous system.

Meprobamate is used in mild anxiety states and as a sedative but is no use in psychoses. It is questionable if meprobamate is superior to a placebo.

Benzodiazepine compounds

These compounds such as chlordiazepoxide, nitrazepam, diazepam, medazepam and oxazepam are mild tranquillizers but are not effective in severe psychoses. They are used to treat anxiety, to relax skeletal muscle, and to combat alcoholism. Diazepam is also given intravenously as a premedication for minor surgery (see page 220), and is an effective anticonvulsant (page 204).

The benzodiazepines do not appear to alter the levels of the brain amines but may act upon the limbic system which governs the complex external manifestations of emotion and upon the polysynaptic spinal reflex arcs subserving muscle tone. They are absorbed orally and are slow to reach peak plasma levels and are slowly excreted in the urine.

The benzodiazepines are relatively safe drugs and less toxic than the barbiturates especially in suicidal attempts.

They can cause tiredness and somnolence as well as ataxia, headache, confusion, and vertigo especially in the elderly. They are also liable to drug misuse (page 236) and to cause dependence. They may also stimulate the appetite and cause obesity.

Other tranquillizers and anxiolytic drugs

There are numerous other drugs which have been used for this purpose. β-adrenergic blocking agents such as propranolol have been shown to be of use to control the sympathetic mediated symptoms of anxiety such as sweating and palpitations.

Benzoctamine resembles the benzodiazepines and may have a low abuse potential. It is thought to act on the gamma efferent fibre system to the skeletal muscle spindle.

ANTIDEPRESSANTS

Drugs which stimulate the central nervous system exist world wide. They range from tea and coffee to more exotic preparations such as the chewing of coca leaves or betel nut. Some drugs may be used therapeutically to relieve depression. Depression is a complex problem and its classification is much disputed. A certain amount of depression is a normal response to traumatic experience (reactive depression) but this may persist and spread to involve every aspect of the patient's life and is often mistaken for organic disease (endogenous depression). A most important part of the treatment is support and reassurance but symptomatic drug therapy is often useful.

Antidepressant drugs may be amphetamine-like sympathomimetic drugs which are primarily stimulants (psychostimulants) or drugs such as the monoamine oxidase inhibitors and imipramine-like drugs which seem to be fairly selective antidepressant drugs (psychic energizers; thymoleptics).

1. Amphetamine and related compounds (see also page 66)

The drugs elevate mood, delay the onset of mental and physical fatigue, and produce marked stimulation which leads to their abuse as 'pep pills'.

(a) *Amphetamine*. This is a sympathomimetic amine (page 62) and a racemic base. It is stable and may be taken by mouth. It is readily absorbed and penetrates to the brain. It is not destroyed by monoamine oxidase or catechol-o-methyl transferase but is destroyed by the microsomal system of the liver, or excreted unchanged in the urine.

Amphetamine has peripheral α- and β-adrenergic actions due to the release of catecholamines which causes stimulation of the heart, a rise in blood pressure, bronchodilatation and inhibition of peristalsis.

Amphetamine has a powerful stimulant action on the central nervous system and lowers the threshold for arousal of the ascending reticular system. This results in increased activity, elevation of mood and improved performance of some tasks. Learning, as such, does not seem to be improved and the beneficial effects on performance may be due to the influence on mood and inclination.

Amphetamine is used for its central stimulant action in the treatment of depression; to overcome temporarily the effects of fatigue; and has been used to treat poisoning by depressant drugs. Amphetamine also causes a reduction in voluntary food intake and so is used as supportive therapy in the treatment of obesity though related compounds such as phenmetrazine and fenfluramine are preferable.

Amphetamine and the amphetamine-like drugs can give rise to psychic dependence (page 238). More acute toxic effects include signs of sympathetic overstimulation and a transitory psychotic reaction.

(b) *Dexamphetamine*. This is the dextro isomer of amphetamine and is 3–4 times as potent as the laevo isomer. It has similar actions to amphetamine though with proportionately stronger central actions.

(c) *Methylamphetamine*. This has central stimulant and peripheral adrenergic actions. It will raise a depressed blood pressure and, though less powerful than noradrenaline, it is not so readily inactivated and so has a more prolonged action.

(d) *Methylphenindate, phenmetrazine.* These also have amphetamine-like actions.

(e) *Tranylcypromine.* This drug is an inhibitor of monoamine oxidase and is related to amphetamine.

(f) *Amphetamine-barbiturate mixtures.* In these mixtures the barbiturate is intended to suppress untoward amphetamine excitement. In certain proportions the mixture causes potentiation of effect and produces great elevation of mood. They are popular as 'pep pills' (e.g. Drinamyl or Purple Hearts, a mixture of amphetamine and amylobarbitone).

2. Monoamine oxidase inhibitors (MAOI)

Monoamine oxidase (MAO) degrades intracellular biogenic amines such as the catecholamines and 5-hydroxytryptamine, and is found in most tissues in the mitochondrial fraction (page 60).

The monoamine oxidase inhibitors (MAOI) block the action of MAO but the relationship between this inhibition and the therapeutic action is not firmly established. There are several natural MAO and the clinically used MAOI also interfere with the degradation of barbiturates, cocaine, pethidine and morphine but not that of histamine.

Chemically the monoamine oxidase inhibitors may be classified as the hydrazine derivatives (iproniazid, isocarboxazid, nialamide, phenelzine), and the non-hydrazine derivatives (especially those related to amphetamine such as tranylcypromine and pargyline).

They were originally discovered when it was found that tuberculous patients treated with isoniazid had elevations of mood not due to a cure of their disease.

They are readily absorbed and quickly excreted, but their action is slow in onset and may be prolonged due to permanent inactivation of the enzyme, so their effect may persist for several weeks after discontinuance of therapy.

The monoamine oxidase inhibitors consequently have very complex pharmacological actions:

(a) *Central nervous system.* They elevate the mood of the depressed patient but may take some weeks to act.

(b) *Cardiovascular system*. They have a hypotensive action similar to sympathetic block. They also give symptomatic relief in angina perhaps due to decreased work because of the fall in blood pressure. Elevation of mood could also play a part and might be dangerous if the patient was no longer careful of observing the limits of his exercise tolerance.

Toxicity. The MAOI may cause excessive central nervous stimulation characterized by tremors, restlessness, anxiety, insomnia and even convulsions.

Postural hypotension may occur, but hypertensive attacks have been reported. These attacks of hypertension usually follow the ingestion of such food as fermented cheese, hung game, beer, yeast, Bovril, Marmite which contain active amines such as tyramine which release catecholamines from the nerve-ending stores. Normally, tyramine is rapidly destroyed by MAO but, if this is inhibited, enough catecholamine may be released to cause large rises of blood pressure. Broad beans contain DOPA (page 58) and similarly may provoke hypertensive reactions.

The action of injected catecholamines is also potentiated but, as these are also broken down by catechol-o-methyl-transferase (which is not affected by MAOI) the effect will not be so great as with ingested tyramine.

Autonomic side effects are similar to ganglion block and include difficulties with micturition, constipation, dry mouth, blurred vision, impotence, and delay in ejaculation.

A serious side effect of the MAOI is the production of hepato-cellular damage and severe jaundice. It occurs especially with the hydrazine derivatives (1/4000 with iproniazid).

The MAOI also enhance the action of barbiturates, general anaesthetics, pethidine and other narcotics. This potentiation persists for at least two weeks after stopping the MAOI.

Uses of MAOI. They are used mainly in the treatment of depression, phobic anxiety states and as antihypertensives. The frequency of adverse reactions does not make them drugs of first choice and it is important that patients are fully instructed as to the possible dangers of food and drug interactions.

. The tricyclic antidepressants (dibenzazepine compounds)

These are related to the phenothiazine derivatives (page 226) but in the iminodibenzyl group (imipramine, desipramine) the connecting sulphur is replaced by an ethylene link and in the dibenzocycloheptadiene group (amitriptyline, nortriptyline, protriptyline) the nitrogen has been replaced by a carbon.

They may be classified according to their different clinical actions. Some such as amitriptyline and trimipramine are sedative and anxiolytic, some such as protriptyline, desipramine and nortriptyline are stimulating with a drive increasing action. Imipramine is not itself an antidepressant but loses a methyl group to become desipramine which is the pharmacologically active substance.

The tricyclic antidepressants are well absorbed orally but their pharmacology is ill understood. Those with stimulant actions appear to preferentially inhibit the re-uptake of noradrenaline whereas others preferentially inhibit the re-uptake of 5-HT. There may be a delay of several weeks before the clinical effects become apparent and care should be taken when the dosage is altered.

The toxic effects of the tricyclic antidepressants are mainly due to the interference with noradrenaline uptake in sympathetic nerve terminals and to their atropine-like action. They include a dry mouth, constipation, dizziness, sweating, tachycardia, palpitations, blurred vision and urinary retention. Other toxic effects are the production of manic symptoms, orthostatic hypotension obstructive jaundice. They also interact with the MAOI to potentiate their effects. Various allergic and hypersensitivity reactions may also occur.

PSYCHODYSLEPTICS

The generic name for these drugs is confused. They are called hallucinogenic because they produce hallucinations, but this name is not always correct as sometimes these are not true hallucinations and can be distinguished from reality. They produce psychotic symptoms and so have been called psychotomimetic but, as the symptoms may be more original than to merely mimic known psychoses, perhaps psychotogenic would be a better term. They have also been called psychedelic drugs to suggest that unsuspected capacities of the imagination may be revealed during the perceptual changes induced by the drug.

The principal hallucinogenic drugs are lysergic acid diethyla mide (LSD), mescaline, psilocybin, psilocin, dimethyltryptamine, marihuana and bufotenine. They have a similar structure as the indole ring is common, save in mescaline which is structurally more akin to adrenaline and noradrenaline. The indole ring is also present in 5-HT, and some relationship between these drugs and 5-HT may account for the hallucinogenic effects. It has also given rise to the hypothesis that schizophrenia results from an error in the metabolism of 5-HT and noradrenaline which produces hallucinogenic substances. This is not yet proven.

LSD and similar drugs have been used therapeutically for the treatment of various psychiatric disorders such as alcoholism, neuroses and psychoses, but there is no great evidence to show beneficial effects.

1. *Lysergic acid diethylamide* (*LSD*–25). Lysergic acid is the common nucleus of the ergot alkaloids (page 95).

Lysergic acid diethylamide is an extremely potent hallucinogen, and as little as 50 μg causes marked disturbances in mood and perception lasting some 8–10 hours, which depend markedly on the dosage, environment, and the basic personality of the individual. These changes are characterized by loss of contact with the environment; distortion of the time sense; phantasies; and hallucinations. These may be very complex and involve cross linking of the senses and, for example, auditory stimuli may produce visual hallucinations.

There are also some objective changes in the peripheral autonomic and central nervous systems which include dilatation of the pupil, increase in blood glucose, and increase in spinal reflexes.

LSD may also cause specific chromosome abnormalities and this is also believed to occur in children born of mothers taking the drug.

LSD is readily absorbed from the gut, though can be given parenterally. It is extensively bound to plasma protein and converted in the liver to non-hallucinogenic metabolites, and only small amounts appear unchanged in the urine and faeces. There is no preferential accumulation in the brain and its mode of action is unknown. It antagonizes 5-HT but other 5-HT antagonists do not produce hallucinations and some hallucinogens do not antagonize 5-HT.

2. *Mescaline*. This is obtained from a Mexican cactus (the tops are peyote or cactus buttons). Mescaline is similar in

structure to the sympathomimetic amines and, as well as causing sympathomimetic effects, produces hallucinations and distortion of the sense of time and space.

It is well absorbed by mouth and is concentrated in the kidneys, liver and spleen and is excreted mainly unchanged.

3. *Psilocin, psilocybin*. These drugs are related substances, and are obtained from a Mexican mushroom. They have hallucinogenic effects which are much less potent than those of LSD and last for 2–4 hours.

4. *Marihuana*. This is a derivative of hemp (Cannabis) and is a mild hallucinogen.

Drug dependence of the hallucinogen type. These drugs may cause drug dependence of a type discussed on page 239.

DRUG DEPENDENCE

There are many drugs that, when taken by some individuals, produce in them a satisfying reaction which persuades them to continue the use of the drug. This can result in drug abuse which is defined as '. . . persistent or sporadic excessive drug use inconsistent with or unrelated to acceptable medical practice . . .' (WHO, 1969).

Drug abuse has two major aspects; that of the effect of the drug on the particular individual and the interplay of drug abuse and society.

It has been customary to divide regular or continuous drug abuse into addiction and habituation though it is not always possible to draw a firm distinction between them. In 1964 the World Health Organisation Expert Committee on Addiction-producing Drugs recommended that the term drug dependence be used instead. Drug dependence may be defined as '. . . a state, psychic and sometimes also physical, resulting from the interaction between a living organism and a drug, characterized by behavioural and other responses that always include a compulsion to take the drug on a continuous or periodic basis in order to experience its psychic effects, and sometimes to avoid the discomfort of its absence. Tolerance may or may not be present. A person may be dependent on more than one drug . . .'. (WHO 1969).

The characteristics of drug dependence vary with the drug

involved but there are three basic phenomena which may occur singly or in combination.

(a) *Psychic dependence* (*emotional dependence*). This is a state of mind in which, although there may be no physical need to take the drug, emotional disturbances result if it is withheld. It is a potent factor with many drugs and may cause intense craving and compulsive abuse.

(b) *Physical dependence*. This is a state in which the organism had adapted at cell level to the drug which has become necessary for normal metabolism to continue. If the drug is withheld, or the body concentration falls below a certain level, or if a specific antagonist is given, an abstinence or withdrawal syndrome results, characteristic of each drug type. These symptoms are relieved by administration of the drug or a similar one.

(c) *Tolerance*. Here an increasing amount of drug is necessary to produce the same effect. It need not affect all actions of the drug to the same degree and may occur with drugs that do not induce physical dependence. There can be cross tolerance to other drugs of the same or different types.

Types of drug dependence

The World Health Organisation recommended that drug dependence be specified by the type of drug involved.

1. *Morphine type*. Tolerance and physical dependence may occur within a day or so of frequent administration of morphine, even with the dose ranges used for therapeutic purposes. This is important to remember in postoperative care.

Morphine dependence is characterized by a strong psychic dependence with an early and increasing physical dependence and tolerance. Four grammes daily may be taken by the addict (normal adult dose is 10–20 mg) who becomes exceptionally tolerant to the depressant, but not all the stimulant actions, with cross tolerance to related drugs and pethidine.

The withholding of the drug or the administration of an antagonist like nalorphine produces a typical withdrawal syndrome which can also happen in a baby born of a dependent mother. The first few symptoms of mild distress with rhinorrhoea and lacrimation pass within 24 hours into an acute insomnia with aches, pains, and hot and cold sensations. Restlessness, vomiting diarrhoea, painful cramps, general malaise and subjective distress reach a peak in 72 hours and then decline though residual symptoms persist for days or weeks.

In treatment, it is usual to cover the withdrawal period with drugs such as methadone, codeine, chlorpromazine and barbiturates. Maintenance of fluid balance and psychotherapy are also essential. Other morphine-like drugs have drug dependence characteristics similar to morphine itself, with some differences depending on their potency and duration of action.

2. *Barbiturate-alcohol type.* Psychic dependence, physical dependence and tolerance occur with the barbiturates and are very similar to those of alcohol, and partial cross dependence results. Chronic users show signs of intoxication such as depression, tremor, ataxia, and social errors. Withdrawal symptoms may be severe with anxiety, tremors, psychotic episodes, and a craving for the drug which begins in 24 hours and takes a week or more to pass off.

This dependence results from many factors, and is mainly present in older age groups. With barbiturates, it may result from misguided prolonged therapeutic use developing into a panacea for emotional disorders. Alcohol dependence may be said to exist when the consumption of alcohol by a person exceeds the limits set by his culture. It is complicated by the emotional problems of the addict and the rules of his particular society.

3. *Amphetamine type.* Tolerance and psychic dependence may result with amphetamine-like drugs, but there does not seem to be a true physical dependence or characteristic withdrawal syndrome. Prolonged use may cause paranoid symptoms similar to schizophrenia.

Barbiturate-amphetamine mixtures have achieved much notoriety as pep pills in adolescent and young people, though a large placebo factor seems to occur.

4. *Cannabis type.* Cannabis (hashish, Indian hemp, kif, dagga, marihuana) is commonly taken by smoking 'pot' or 'reefers' and induces a dream-like state with alterations of consciousness and perception. Hallucinations and disorientation may result. Cannabis causes slight tolerance with no physical dependence, though psychic dependence may be strong. The active principle, tetrahydrocannabinol, has been isolated.

5. *Cocaine type.* Cocaine dependence is common in Indians of

the high Andes who chew coca leaves to relieve cold, fatigue and hunger. It has the reputation of stimulating sexual desires and causes euphoria, hallucinations and paranoid delusions. It is commonly taken as snuff ('snow') which may ulcerate the nasal mucosa or perforate the nasal septum. It is also taken by injection, especially intravenously. Psychic dependence may be marked though there seems not to be physical dependence or tolerance.

6. *Hallucinogen type*. Drugs such as LSD, psilocybin and mescaline can be the source of psychic dependence, though this is usually not marked and not associated with physical dependence, Considerable tolerance to LSD develops but on stopping the drug soon goes. There is cross-tolerance between LSD, mescaline, and psilocybin. These drugs can also produce variable periods of psychosis which may recur intermittently for a long period.

REFERENCES

Poldinger, W. (1967) *Compendium of Psychopharmacology*. Basle: Roche.

World Health Organisation. Technical Report Series. Geneva: WHO.

(*a*) No. 407 (1969) WHO Expert Committee on Drug Dependence. 16th Report.

(*b*) No. 273 (1964) WHO Expert Committee on Addiction Producing Drugs. 13th Report.

(*c*) No. 371 (1967) Research in Psychopharmacology.

Local anaesthetics (local analgesics) block conduction along the axon and can prevent sense organs from initiating afferent impulses. Suitably administered, they can cause anaesthesia of a region of the body without the loss of consciousness that occurs in general anaesthesia.

The ideal local anaesthetic

This should have a specific and reversible action upon sensory nerves and act topically (i.e. on body surfaces). It should have a rapid onset of action with adequate duration; with low systemic toxicity, and cause no hypersensitivity. It should be water soluble, stable in solution, and allow of combination with adrenaline.

Mode of action of local anaesthetics

Most local anaesthetics, procaine for example, are tertiary amine esters of an aromatic acid such as para-amino benzoic acid and are hence weak bases. There are exceptions, however, as lignocaine is an anilide derivative and cinchocaine is a quinoline derivative, which may be useful if sensitization develops to the tertiary amine esters.

Many other drugs having parasympatholytic, antihistaminic, tranquillizing or quinidine-like properties are also amine esters of an aromatic acid and have local anaesthetic properties. However, tissue irritation or other effects stops them being used as local anaesthetics.

Local anaesthetics are usually administered as the acid salts which are stable and water soluble. These must hydrolyse in the tissues to give the free base which is lipid soluble and probably enters the nerve at the nodes of Ranvier to inactivate sodium transport and stabilize the membrane. Whilst this has little effect on the resting potential of the nerve, depolarization and propagation of the impulse are prevented.

Local anaesthetics can abolish all sensation, but pain fibres are affected first as they are thinner, unmyelinated and so more easily penetrated by the anaesthetic. In higher concentrations of anaesthetic, all nerves will be affected.

Pharmacology of the local anaesthetics

Many local anaesthetics (but not procaine) are absorbed from mucous membranes and are destroyed mainly in the liver and by plasma esterases.

The local anaesthetics have other actions than that of nerve block. These actions are responsible for the toxic effects which occur especially if the rate of absorption exceeds the rate of elimination. One must therefore take into account the patient's age, weight, physique, clinical condition, the presence of liver damage, the site of injection and the amount of the particular drug used. Intravenous administration is especially dangerous, though some local anaesthetics, such as cocaine, are absorbed from mucous membranes with comparable speed. Absorption from inflamed tissues may also be so rapid as to cause systemic effects.

The central nervous system may be stimulated to cause anxiety, restlessness, tremors and convulsions, and this stimulation may eventually lead to medullary depression and death.

A quinidine-like action on the heart may cause myocardial depression and bradycardia (see procainamide, page 145). Smooth muscle is relaxed and neuromuscular conduction is depressed due to a curare-like action.

Hypersensitivity may become a problem with the local anaesthetics and is prone to occur in those handling them regularly, such as medical and dental staff.

Methods of using local anaesthetics

Local anaesthesia may be produced by methods other than paralysing sensory nerve endings with drugs. Some of these methods are obsolete, such as by pressure on nerve trunks or by tissue ischaemia with a tourniquet, though others, such as the application of cold (ethyl chloride, refrigeration), are still used.

The local anaesthetics may be required to have prolonged effects. Giving them as depot solutions in wax or oil is not very effective. The use of vasoconstrictor drugs such as adrenaline prolongs their action by decreasing their absorption. Vasoconstrictor drugs also decrease the incidence of toxic effects of the local anaesthetics, as these depend on blood concentration of the drug, which is less when absorption is slow as this allows more time for metabolic degradation. Adrenaline in excess may produce ischaemic necrosis of the injection site and should not be present in local anaesthetic used to anaesthetize digits. Adrenaline may also cause systemic toxic effects and is usually not given in higher concentrations than 1/200000 and not more than a total of 0·5 mg. Dentists use a 1/80000 dilution.

Prolonged local anaesthesia (e.g. of the trigeminal nerve in trigeminal neuralgia) can be produced by the injection of phenol or alcohol which causes death of the tissue.

Local anaesthetics may be applied to mucous membranes especially of the eye, nose, throat, urethra, and bladder (topical application). Other tissues may be anaesthetized by blocking the nerves supplying the part (regional or conduction anaesthesia), or by injecting the drug locally into the tissue (infiltration anaesthesia). It is also possible to introduce the drug into the subarachnoid or intrathecal space (spinal anaesthesia) to block the posterior nerve roots. By selection of the site of injection, position of the patient, and specific gravity of the anaesthetic solution (which can rise or fall among the nerve roots), it is possible to get some degree of selectivity in spinal anaesthesia. In epidural anaesthesia, the anaesthetic is given into the epidural space; a useful technique in obstetric practice.

Individual local anaesthetics

1. *Cocaine.* Cocaine is an alkaloid obtained from *Erythroxylon coca* and is the benzoyl methyl ester of ecgonine. Cocaine is well

absorbed from mucous membranes and can rapidly cause toxic effects; though as it potentiates adrenaline (page 70), the ensuing vasoconstriction lessens the absorption.

Cocaine is a stimulant of the central nervous system especially the cortex and causes motor excitement, increased wakefulness and endurance to hunger and cold. The chewing of coca leaves by South American natives for this purpose is well known. Cocaine is also a drug of dependence but this is discussed elsewhere (page 238).

If instilled into the conjunctival sac, cocaine causes anaesthesia, blanching of the sclera, dilatation of the pupil and retraction of the upper lid.

Cocaine is now used solely as a surface anaesthetic for mucosal and conjunctival surfaces and, because of its toxicity, is no longer used as an infiltration anaesthetic.

2. *Procaine.* Procaine is an ester of para-amino benzoic acid. It is poorly absorbed from mucous membranes and has to be injected and so is of no value as a surface anaesthetic. Procaine is rapidly hydrolysed by procaine esterases (probably pseudo-cholinesterase) to give para-amino benzoic acid and diethylaminoethanol. It is a vasodilator and not a vasoconstrictor and is usually given with adrenaline.

Procaine has muscle relaxant and quinidine-like actions (see also procainamide, page 145). It is much less toxic than cocaine, though this depends to a large extent on its poor absorption. Toxic effects include convulsions, respiratory paralysis, hypotension, and skin sensitization. Procaine is used mainly for infiltration and conduction anaesthesia.

3. *Lignocaine.* Lignocaine is not an ester but an anilide derivative, and is therefore not destroyed by plasma esterase. It is not a vasodilator or vasoconstrictor and is rapidly absorbed from mucous membranes. The onset of action is rapid and lasts for an hour or so, though this is greatly prolonged by the addition of adrenaline.

The toxicity of lignocaine is similar to procaine, but as it is more potent ($\times 2\frac{1}{2}$), the therapeutic ratio is better. Lignocaine is used for infiltration, nerve trunk, or topical anaesthesia.

4. *Prilocaine.* This is similar in potency to lignocaine but may be less toxic.

5. *Bupivicaine.* This drug is related to lignocaine and is four

244 PHARMACOLOGY

times as potent. It causes a prolonged local anaesthesia of 8–15 hours duration.

6. *Amethocaine*. This is very effective both topically and by injection. It is very potent and rapidly absorbed and can easily cause toxic effects.

7. *Benzocaine*. This has low toxicity and potency. It is used topically to relieve pain or irritation in the mouth, pharynx, or around the anus.

REFERENCES

Bromage, P. R. (1966) *The Mechanism of Action of Local Anaesthetics*. Berlin: Springer Verlag.

Wiedling, S. & Tegnér, C. (1963) Local anaesthetics. In *Progress in Medicinal Chemistry*, 3, 332. Ellis, G. P. & West, G. B. (eds.). London: Butterworth.

The oral route of administration is of great importance and has been dealt with on page 7. Many drugs, however, are given for their local effect on the gastrointestinal tract; usually to depress or stimulate secretions or motility.

GASTRIC SECRETION

Gastric juice has a high concentration of hydrogen and chloride ions which provide the optimal pH of 1·5–4 for pepsin to act, and secretion is controlled by both nervous and humoral factors. Stimulation of the vagus, directly or reflexly, increases gastric secretion which may also be increased by the action of gastrin.

Gastrin. This hormone is secreted from the antral region of the stomach in response to the presence of food. It is a peptide of 17 residues and there are two forms, gastrin I and gastrin II (which differs from gastrin I only by sulphonation of tyrosine residue). Gastrin stimulates the flow of a pepsin-free acid juice but, in higher doses, it inhibits acid secretion and stimulates the secretion of pepsin and pancreatic juices. Gastrin also increases the mobility of the fundus and jejunum.

Pentagastrin. This synthetic compound contains 5 amino acids but still has gastrin-like action and may be used to test gastric secretory capacity.

ANTACIDS

A common aim of modifying gastric function is to treat peptic ulcer and other forms of dyspepsia. There is a traditional belief that indigestion is due to gastric 'acid', though there seems to be no constant relationship between the pain of a peptic ulcer and the level of gastric acidity, but the neutralization of gastric acid does give symptomatic relief.

It is not easy to diminish the acidity of the gastric juice by reducing the secretion of acid, though some drugs will do this. It is easier to neutralize the acid directly.

The ideal antacid

This would not be absorbed and so not likely to disturb the acid–base balance. It would be rapid in action with a prolonged effect and not prone to cause diarrhoea, constipation, acid rebounds, or eructation.

Unfortunately, the antacids in therapeutic use are not ideal and many have undesirable side effects.

Types of antacid

Antacids may be classified in several ways. Systemic antacids are those which can be absorbed and so change the acid–base balance, whereas non-systemic antacids are not absorbed and are unlikely to change the acid–base balance. Perhaps a better classification is to consider whether antacids act as chemical neutralizers or as physical adsorbents of acid. Those drugs acting on the central nervous system to prevent secretion of acid should also be included.

1. *Sodium bicarbonate.* This is a very popular systemic antacid, taken alone or in a mixture. It rapidly neutralizes stomach acid with the production of carbon dioxide and sodium chloride. The carbon dioxide can cause noisy eructations which may cause satisfaction to the patient.

Any excess base is absorbed and could cause alkalosis and the secretion of an alkaline urine. Theoretically, at least, it is possible to overneutralize and cause an acid rebound. Prolonged use is not only likely to cause chronic alkalaemia but may also lower the renal threshold to glucose and cause glycosuria.

2. *Magnesium hydroxide* (*Milk of Magnesia*). This is an insoluble powder which reacts with hydrochloric acid to form magnesium chloride with no evolution of carbon dioxide. Very

little chloride is lost and there is no danger of alkalosis, but residual soluble and unabsorbed magnesium compounds may act as a saline purge. Magnesium oxide is a widely used antacid converted in water to the hydroxide and so has similar properties.

3. *Magnesium carbonate*. This has similar antacid properties to magnesium hydroxide, but carbon dioxide is liberated during the neutralization of stomach acid.

4. *Magnesium trisilicate*. Magnesium trisilicate, a salt of meso-trisilic acid, functions as a non-systematic antacid. It is an insoluble powder which reacts slowly over several hours with hydrochloric acid to form magnesium chloride and colloidal silica. The colloidal silica also directly adsorbs acid. In the relatively neutral small intestine, magnesium trisilicate is reformed, hence there is a buffering action which avoids loss of chloride.

5. *Aluminium salts*. Aluminium hydroxide, a mixture of the hydroxide and the hydrated oxide, both adsorbs acid and directly neutralizes it to form aluminium chloride. It is slow in action, not absorbed, and may inactivate pepsin by a direct action. It is liable to cause constipation, and, by forming insoluble phosphates, may cause phosphate deficiency. It may be preferable to use aluminium phosphate which, though not so powerful an antacid, will not cause phosphate deficiency.

Aluminium glycinate is aluminium hydroxide combined with glycine and gives good buffering with no danger of alkalosis.

6. *Calcium salts*. These include calcium hydroxide and calcium carbonate. As they are constipating, they are often given in combination with magnesium salts, which are laxative.

Other drugs used in the treatment of peptic ulceration

1. *Anticholinergic drugs*. Drugs such as atropine and hyoscine may reduce gastric secretion and are of use in the treatment of peptic ulceration (pages 50, 97). Newer anticholinergic drugs include oxyphencyclimine, a tertiary amine acting at the post-ganglionic effector site and quaternary ammonium salts such as propantheline. The clinical use of these drugs is limited by their actions on other cholinergically innervated organs though various of them are claimed to have some selectivity of action.

2. *Liquorice derivatives*. The mode of action of these substances in healing duodenal and gastric ulceration is not known but is

probably due to increased mucus secretion which protects the gastric cells and to an increased cell turnover which promotes epithelialization of damaged areas. Crude liquorice has two active principles, a 'spasmolytic agent' which is as yet undefined and glycyrrhizin, a derivative of glycyrrhetinic acid (enoxolone), each of which is available more or less separately.

Carbenoxolone. This substance is a triterpene synthesized from glycyrrhetinic acid. It has anti-inflammatory properties probably due to stimulation of endogenous corticosteroid production. Carbenoxolone is useful in the treatment of gastric ulcer but its corticosteroid effects may cause hypertension, hypokalaemia and impaired glucose tolerance.

3. *Various drugs.* Other drugs used in the treatment of peptic ulceration include gefarnate, carragenins which are anti-pepsin substances extracted from seaweed as well as various tranquillizing and antidepressive drugs.

ANTI-EMETICS

Vomiting is primarily a protective action to rid the stomach of noxious substances, but may also result from any kind of sensation especially labrynthine or emotional. Vomiting associated with travel, pregnancy, surgery, or the administration of drugs can be a great problem.

Vomiting is controlled by a vomiting centre in the lateral reticular formation with a trigger zone in the area postrema, though other areas such as the cerebellum may be involved. This complexity of pathways, and the different modes of action of various causes of vomiting, may explain why some drugs are effective in one kind of vomiting but not in another.

Many drugs cause vomiting either by a direct irritant action on the stomach or by a central action. Drugs acting centrally usually act on the trigger zone and include digitalis, apomorphine, veratrum, cytotoxic drugs and radiation. Save for apomorphine, they are not used for this purpose.

Therapeutically, it is usually necessary to stop vomiting rather than to cause it; but, if needed, vomiting may be produced acutely by a finger poked inside the patient's throat. A somewhat less heroic method is to give a strong sodium chloride solution.

Drug-induced vomiting, radiation sickness and post-operative vomiting may be successfully treated by the phenothiazine derivatives such as chlorpromazine and perphenazine (page 226).

Motion sickness. This may be produced by any form of travel, and whilst being mainly labyrinthine in origin, is also complicated by visual, olfactory, and emotional factors.

Hyoscine (page 51) is the most effective drug, though complicated by the side effects of dry mouth and blurred vision if given in adequate amounts. Many antihistamines such as meclozine and cyclizine (page 89) are also effective. These drugs may cause drowsiness and may potentiate the action of alcohol and hypnotic drugs. Patients should be warned against these dangerous side effects especially if they intend to drive or use moving machinery.

Vomiting in pregnancy. This is common from the first month of pregnancy (morning sickness) though tends to pass off after the fifth month. The treatment is complicated by the possibility of drug-induced fetal abnormality and some argue that no drug should be used in early pregnancy unless in extreme urgency.

Various trials, however, have shown that meclozine and cyclizine produce no apparent increased risk of teratogeneticity, and are effective. Other drugs such as promethazine, promethazine theoclate, and diphenhydramine have been used for many years without suspicion that they are teratogenetic. Pyridoxine has also been used and, whilst entirely safe, is of dubious effectiveness.

It is probably best to treat morning sickness with one of these compounds rather than with newer and untried drugs. It might also be advisable to restrict treatment to patients where vomiting is seriously interfering with normal life.

PURGATIVES

This term is usually taken to be synonymous with laxative, cathartic, aperient and evacuant and includes drugs which are taken to cause defaecation. They are not of exceptional therapeutic importance save in the lay mind of a need to keep the bowels open. They are used to treat constipation (a vague term); to clear the bowel preoperatively or after some antihelminthics, and to aid in the induction of labour.

Constipation, which in the acute form may be symptomatic of acute intestinal obstruction, is usually taken to mean the infrequent passage of stools, but what is infrequent is arguable and stools may quite normally be passed several times a day or only once every 2–3 days. In the treatment of chronic constipation, retraining to heed the physiological call to defaecation and a high residue diet are often successful.

Purgatives may act by a bulk effect, by a lubricant (emollient) effect, or by irritation.

Bulk purgatives

The presence of bulky substances in the gut stimulates peristalsis and promotes defaecation. Fruit and vegetables contain cellulose which is not digested and will provide roughage. Some fruits, such as prunes and figs, also contain stimulant purgatives. Bran is commonly taken as a cereal and contains a lot of indigestible fibres.

Some substances, such as methyl cellulose, agar, pysllium, and slippery elm contain indigestible substances which, on contact with water, swell up and provide additional bulk.

Saline purges are classically said to act by attracting and retaining fluid in the intestinal lumen by osmosis thereby increasing the bulk of the contents. Recent evidence, however, suggests that the hormone cholecystokininpancreozymin may be released by the saline purge to produce complex motor and secretory effects which account for their observed clinical actions. The saline purges act in 1–3 hours and are given on an empty stomach. Substances used include magnesium sulphate (Epsom Salts), sodium sulphate (Glauber's Salts), and sodium potassium tartrate (Rochelle Salts), which, with sodium bicarbonate and tartaric acid make Seidlitz Powder. Many of the effervescent patent preparations fall in this group.

Lubricant purgatives

Liquid paraffin is an oily inert liquid. Whilst it lubricates and softens the faeces, it also provides extra bulk as it is not digested. It is useful to prevent straining at stool postoperatively or in patients with haemorrhoids or heart disease. The use of liquid paraffin has been linked with polyposis, vitamins D and K deficiency, and inhalation pneumonia.

Glycerin suppositories may also be useful as lubricant purgatives.

Irritant purgatives

These compounds have a local stimulant action on the intestinal wall and excite Auerbach's plexus to cause increased peristalsis. Ideally they should not irritate the stomach, which could cause vomiting, and should produce only a mild irritation of the intestine or griping will occur.

1. *Castor oil*. This is a triglyceride obtained from the seeds of the castor oil plant. The oil is inert and soothing and may be used in the eye but is hydrolysed by lipase in the small intestine to ricinoleic acid, which stimulates the small intestine. It is given on an empty stomach and acts in 2–6 hours.

2. *Phenolphthalein*. This compound stimulates the large intestine and acts in 6–8 hours. Some is absorbed in the small intestine and excreted via the bile and the urine and will cause a red colour if the urine or faeces is alkaline.

3. *Bisacodyl*. This compound stimulates the large intestine in 5–10 hours and may be given by mouth or as suppositories.

4. *The anthracene group (anthraquinone or emodin group)*. This group includes such drugs as cascara, rhubarb, senna and aloes. The active principle, emodin, acts on the large intestine and so reflexly stimulates the small intestine. These purgatives have a somewhat lengthy delay before they act (6–10 hours), as they are first absorbed as an inactive glycoside which is broken down to the active principle emodin which is excreted in the bile and large intestine where it has its action. Senna is used as an infusion of the leaves or pod (senna tea), though is available in a standardized form.

Other purgatives

Many other compounds are used to produce purgation. They include the mercurial salts such as calomel; the drastic purges such as jalap, colocynth and podophyllum; sulphur; liquorice. Their importance is minimal save in their availability to the lay public.

Diarrhoea

Diarrhoea can be caused by serious diseases such as typhoid or dysentery when correct diagnosis and specific treatment is urgently necessary. Often however it is due to ill-defined causes such as a sudden change in diet, bacterial toxins or virus infection and is characterized by sudden explosive diarrhoea running a self limiting course of a few days. The association with travel is reflected by the various local names, Gippy Tummy, Bombay Trots, turista. Chemotherapy of this traveller's diarrhoea is not normally necessary and it can usually be successfully treated symptomatically.

Adsorbents. Mixtures containing charcoal, chalk or kaolin are said to work by adsorption of toxin though this is dubious.

Drugs reducing gut motility. Preparations containing opium type drugs such as codeine or morphine reduce the tone and motility of the bowel. They are often combined with an adsorbent. Diphenoxylate, a pethidine derivative, can also be used and is often combined with atropine.

The fact that certain drugs are toxic to some organisms or tissues but not to others is the rationale of chemotherapy, and a chemotherapeutic agent may be defined as a drug used to kill parasites in a host without harming the host. Chemotherapy includes the treatment of bacterial, virus, protozoal, and helminth infections. The term is also used when speaking of the drug treatment of cancer.

It is customary to distinguish between an antimicrobial drug and an antibiotic. An antimicrobial drug is one used against micro-organisms whereas an antibiotic is more restricted in meaning and is a compound produced by one organism which is toxic to another. As so many antibiotics are now wholly or partially synthesized, strict academic distinction is no longer valid.

MODES OF ACTION OF ANTIMICROBIAL DRUGS

Rational development of chemotherapy requires knowledge of the relationship between the structure of the drug and the site of action in the parasite cell. A parasite grows as a result of organized synthetic activities and a drug may inhibit this synthetic activity or disorganize essential structures. Whilst described here for the bacterial cell, the principles are the same for other kinds of chemotherapy and additional information is given in the relevant chapter.

The bacterial cell has a tough outside wall surrounding the cell membrane to protect it from the deformation that could be caused by the osmotic difference between the cell and its environment. In the cell substance are the synthetic mechanisms controlling metabolism of the cell. Prominent among these is the process of protein replication which involves desoxyribonucleic acid (DNA) and ribonucleic acid (RNA). Interference may therefore be at one or more of several sites:

1. *The cell wall.* This consists of highly polymerized mucopeptides which are long chains of amino sugars with peptide side chains. These side chains are cross linked to give great tensile

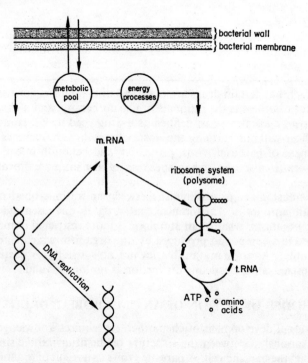

FIG. 13. Possible sites of action of chemotherapeutic agents in the bacterial cell.

strength and rigidity. Some drugs such as penicillin, cephalosporins, bacitracin, vancomycin, and cycloserine inhibit the formation of mucopeptides. When the bacterial cell continues to grow the wall is defective and weak so the cell bursts by osmotic action. This type of drug attacks bacteria which are growing and dividing, as then the cell wall is being constantly formed, and has much less effect on dormant bacteria. The wall mucopeptides are specifically bacterial structures and do not occur in mammalian cells so these drugs are especially selective. Penicillin, for example, blocks the peptide linkage between N-acetylmuramic acid and N-acetyl-glucosamine. These are found in Gram-positive bacteria, but in most Gram-negative bacteria the cell wall composition is different and they are insensitive to penicillin.

2. *The cytoplasmic membrane.* This lipoprotein structure is an osmotic barrier, the site of respiratory enzymes and cytochrome linked electron transport. Compounds such as polymyxin, tyrocidin and gramicidin disorganize the membrane, but their selectivity is low and they act on cells in general and are usually too toxic for systemic use. Nystatin and amphotericin react with sterols in membranes to cause lysis. Sterols are present in the cell membranes of yeasts and fungi but not bacteria. Unfortunately, sterols are also present in the cell membranes of mammals so toxicity is high.

3. *Replication processes.* The complex mechanism of protein synthesis and DNA is very vulnerable to interference. Some compounds may attack DNA either by bridging the strands (actinomycin, mitomycin), or by inserting into the coils (acridine). As a result the helix partially untwists and suffers distortion, so replication and transcription processes are disorganized. These compounds have little selective toxicity and are used in cancer chemotherapy (page 291).

4. *Translation stages of protein synthesis.* Some compounds such as chloramphenicol, tetracyclines, erythromycin and streptomycin become bound to the ribosome and hinder its movement along the strand of messenger-RNA. This prevents formation of peptide bonds and lengthening of the partially formed polypeptides. It may also cause misreading of the genetic code.

The lack of action on mammalian cells has been explained by differences in ribosomal structure, and there is a drug, cyclohexi-mide, which becomes attached to mammalian ribosomes but not to bacterial. Resistance may also be due to differences in permeability of the membrane or of enzymes which degrade the drug.

5. *Antimetabolite action.* Sulphonamides act as competitive antagonists in the formation of folic acid from p-amino benzoic acid (page 260). Many other antimicrobial drugs are metabolic

analogues interfering with normal synthesis. Cycloserine, for example, is an analogue of D-alanine and prevents its incorporation into the cell wall. Puromycin is an analogue of the terminal nucleotide in transfer-RNA and is a non-selective inhibitor of protein synthesis.

Bactericidal drugs. These destroy the organisms directly and act especially if they are dividing rapidly (e.g. penicillin).

Bacteriostatic drugs. These inhibit growth and multiplication and so allow the natural defences to function more efficiently (e.g. tetracyclines).

It is not possible to generalize on the effects of combinations of the two types of drugs, but obviously the action of penicillin depends on the organism being active and will be hindered by a drug which inhibits multiplication.

The use of antimicrobial drugs

Successful chemotherapy must be rational and this demands a clinical and bacteriological diagnosis with the implication that the case of the disease is a particular micro-organism. Chemotherapy is aimed at the micro-organism and not at the disease as such. Many diseases are caused by a single micro-organism and clinical diagnosis of typhoid, typhus or anthrax for example gives an implicit microbic diagnosis. On the other hand, the clinical diagnosis of pneumonia, meningitis, urinary tract infection may be due to a number of different bacteria. Even a single bacteriological diagnosis is not always enough as the susceptibility of different strains of a bacterial species to an antimicrobial drug may vary greatly (see 'drug resistance'). The *in vitro* assessment of bacterial sensitivity should also be viewed with caution as it need not necessarily reflect the interaction of drug, host and parasite. In plain words, the successful use of a chemotherapeutic agent depends upon the answer to the question: 'Can it kill these organisms in this patient at this time?' Obviously, too, the choice of drug is influenced by considerations of toxicity and efficacy relative to other drugs and the severity of the disease. The use of a toxic drug may be obligatory in life threatening disease if it is the only one effective but it should not be used if a less effective but less toxic drug is suitable or in minor diseases.

Antibacterial spectrum. Many parasites are not affected by some chemotherapeutic agents and this natural resistance may be explicable in terms of the selective toxicity and sites of action already discussed. The antibacterial spectrum refers to the range of organisms which a particular drug will normally destroy. Benzylpenicillin, for example, is active mainly against organisms such as the staphylococcus but is inactive against shigella and salmonella. If the range of organisms is wide, the drug is said to be broad (wide) spectrum as opposed to the narrow spectrum of other drugs.

Drug resistance. Apart from this natural resistance, strains of micro-organisms have emerged that are resistant to drugs to which as a species they were formerly sensitive. One reason for the emergence of resistant trains is by spontaneous mutation and proliferation of resistant variants. Resistance may be due to tolerance to the drug by the use of alternative metabolic paths, and indeed in some extreme cases the drug itself may become an essential metabolite. Increased destruction of the drug can result from enzyme induction and penicillin, for example, is rapidly destroyed by penicillinase produced by some forms of staphylococcus.

Another mechanism by which resistant strains may emerge is transferable drug resistance in which a factor (the R factor) is transferred by conjugation from one bacterium to another even of different species or genera. This can affect a wide range of organisms such as escherichia, salmonella, shigella, proteus, vibrio and is most likely to occur in the bowel. It may result in a resistant but non-pathogenic species transferring resistance to a drug to a sensitive and pathogenic species. As the R-factor plasmids (extra-chromosomal particles of genetic material) may carry the determinants for drug resistance for as many as 9 compounds, it will be seen that multiple drug resistance can easily occur. Resistance can also be transferred by transduction of phage (especially in staphylococci of the same group).

Superinfection. The normal saprophytic flora of the intestinal and respiratory tracts exert a watchdog role and oppose colonization by intruders. If they are destroyed (e.g. by broad spectrum antibiotics such as tetracyclines or chloramphenicol), they are replaced by resistant organisms which may be pathogenic and spread rapidly due to the absence of territorial competition. This is especially likely to occur with staphylococcus, pseudomonas, proteus, and candida. They cause symptoms ranging from a mild disturbance of bowel habit to a fulminating, fatal enteritis.

Protein binding. The importance of protein binding of a drug has already been discussed (page 11). Only the free drug is available for diffusion into tissues and total plasma concentrations give no direct indication of the amount of bound and so therapeutically inactive drug.

REFERENCES

Garrod, L. P., Lambert, H. P. & O'Grady, F. (1973) *Antibiotic and Chemotherapy,* 4th edn. Edinburgh: Livingstone.

Hash, I. H. (1972) Antibiotic Mechanisms. *Annual Review of Pharmacology,* **12,** 35–56. Palo Alto: Annual Reviews Inc.

22 Chemotherapy II: Antibacterial, Antifungal and Antiviral Drugs

---

SULPHONAMIDES

The sulphonamides are synthetic antibacterial agents and, though recent advances in chemotherapy have lessened their usefulness, they remain a valuable group of drugs. The basic sulphonamide structure is that of sulphanilamide (see diagram) and the majority of derivatives have substitutions in the amide group. Some do have substitutions in the amino group which, however, results in loss of bacteriostatic properties and the free group must be restored *in vivo*.

amide group $SO_2.NH_2$

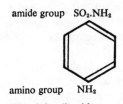

amino group NH_2

(i) sulphanilamide
(*p*-aminobenzene sulphonamide)

COOH

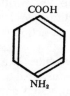

NH_2

(ii) *p*-aminobenzoic acid

The structure of the sulphonamides and *p*-aminobenzoic acid

Some sulphonamides are used for other than antibacterial action. The sulphonylureas (tolbutamide, chlorpropamide) are oral hypoglycaemic agents. Some aromatic and heterocyclic sulphonamides (e.g. acetazolamide, dichlorphenamide) are potent inhibitors of carbonic anhydrase and are used as diuretics.

Mode of action of the sulphonamides

Many bacteria need folic acid for DNA synthesis and obtain it via p-aminobenzoic acid (PABA) (see diagram). This is very similar to the basic structure of sulphonamides which act as competitive antagonists or antimetabolites in the transformation of p-aminobenzoic acid to folic (dihydrofolic) acid under the influence of tetrahydropteroic acid synthetase. and so prevent normal reproduction and metabolism of the organism. Sulphonamides are therefore bacteriostatic and toxic only to organisms that synthesize their own folic acid. In man, folic acid has to be preformed and ingested and sulphonamides do not interfere with this.

Pharmacology of the sulphonamides

Most sulphonamides are well absorbed from the gut and distributed throughout the body water including the cerebrospinal fluid. Some sulphonamides (such as succinylsulphathiazole and phthalysulphathiazole) are poorly adsorbed and so are used for gut infections, though systemically active sulphonamides will be better if the infection is in the wall of the gut and not the lumen.

Sulphonamides are protein bound; the percentage varying from 20% with sulphanilamide, 50–80% with sulphadimidine, and up to 98% with the long acting sulphonamides such as sulphamethoxypyridazine. The protein-bound fraction has no antibacterial action (see page 11) as it is not available for diffusion.

Sulphonamides are excreted via the kidney either unchanged or as the acetylated or conjugated metabolite. The rate of elimination varies, and 4 hourly doses may be necessary for sulphathiazole, sulphanilamide and sulphacetamide; 6 hourly doses for sulphadimidine, sulphamerazine and sulphadiazine; and daily doses for sulphamethoxypyridazine. There is little reabsorption from the kidney tubules and the urine concentration is high.

Antibacterial actions of the sulphonamides

The various types differ little in individual specificity against bacteria. They have a wide antibacterial spectrum and are effective against most of the major Gram-positive and Gram-negative pathogenic bacteria.

Toxic effects of the sulphonamides

Most of these are mild, such as nausea, malaise, headache, cyanosis (due to methaemoglobinaemia). Localized application can cause photosensitization, with the production of eczema on exposure to sunlight.

More serious complications include crystalluria where the relatively insoluble acetyl derivative is deposited in the kidney and may cause loss of renal function. The risk of crystalluria is lessened by the use of more soluble sulphonamides such as sulphadimidine and sulphafurazole; by making the urine alkaline, and by increasing the volume of the urine.

Other serious complications are those of hypersensitivity, depression of the bone marrow, and agranulocytosis.

Individual sulphonamides

1. *Sulphadimidine.* This is the best routine sulphonamide. It is rapidly absorbed and fairly soluble in the urine and needs to be given every 4–6 hours. It is especially useful in meningococcal meningitis, though sulphadiazine may penetrate better to the cerebrospinal fluid. It is also useful in *Esch. coli* infections of the urinary tract and in pneumococcal pneumonia.

2. *Pthalylsulphathiazole.* This sulphonamide is poorly absorbed and may be used in the treatment of bacillary dysentery. Sulphaguanidine and succinylsulphathiazole are similar.

3. *Sulphamethoxypyridazine.* This is a long-acting drug and needs to be given once a day only. Much of it is protein bound and so therapeutically inactive and there is no unequivocal evidence of its superiority.

4. *Sulphacetamide sodium.* This may be used in the treatment of some eye infections. It is available as eye drops or ointment.

5. *Sulphasalazine.* This is a compound of salicyclic acid and sulphapyridine. Its major use is in ulcerative colitis to prevent relapse after an acute attack.

Trimethoprim–sulphamethoxazole (co-trimoxazole)

Trimethoprim (see page 279) inhibits dihydrofolate reductase and so prevents reduction of dihydrofolic acid to folinic (tetrahydrofolic acid). Although this is also an essential step in human metabolism, trimethoprim is some ten to a hundred thousand times more active on the bacterial enzyme and so can seriously disrupt their production of DNA and RNA without harming their human host. When trimethoprim is given in combination with sulphamethoxazole, a typical sulphonamide which (page 260) prevents the conversion of PABA to dihydrofolic acid, 2 sequential metabolic steps in the bacterium are thus affected. The combination is probably truly bactericidal unlike the bacteriostatic effects of the individual drugs and may also show true potentiation of effect (page 22).

The ratio used is fixed as 1:5 of trimethoprim and sulphamethoxazole and the latter was chosen as having a similar half life to trimethoprim. The combination has especial value in the treatment of urinary tract infections and secondary infective episodes of chronic bronchitis (especially when due to *H. influenza*) Side effects are similar to those of the sulphonamides.

PENICILLINS

This is the name given to a group of antibiotics originating from work done by Fleming, who in 1928, noticed that a mould, *Penicillium notatum*, was causing lysis of a culture plate of staphylococci. The active substance, which he called penicillin, was so unstable that it was not until 1940 that Florey and Chain managed to isolate enough for a therapeutic trial. The mechanization of production on a vast commercial scale by the U.S.A in World War Two is a matter of history.

Several different strains of *Penicillium* are now used and by feeding various substrates, different penicillins are formed. The penicillin nucleus (6–aminopenicillanic acid) has been isolated and can be modified to give a whole family of semisynthetic penicillins.

Mode of action of the penicillins. They are bactericidal and interfere with cell wall synthesis and are maximally effective against rapidly multiplying organisms. This action is discussed on page 254.

Benzylpenicillin (soluble penicillin; penicillin G)

Benzylpenicillin is the major naturally occurring penicillin and its potency is expressed either in terms of weight of the pure material or in terms of specific antibacterial activity of a reference standard.

Benzylpenicillin is rapidly absorbed from the gut but is inactivated to a major degree by stomach acid and is not very effective by mouth. It is rapidly absorbed parenterally and distributed throughout the body but does not pass readily into the cerebrospinal fluid unless the meninges are inflamed. Benzylpenicillin is rapidly excreted via the urine mainly unchanged, though some is degraded to penicilloic acid. Not only is it filtered at the glomerulus but is also actively secreted by the kidney tubules, and some 60% of an injected dose appears in the urine within 2 hours.

Benzylpenicillin is usually given intramuscularly as the sodium or potassium salt (Benzylpenicillin Injection B.P.); and other routes such as local application are not advisable as they may lead to sensitization.

Benzylpenicillin has three major disadvantages:

1. *Rapid absorption and excretion.* Administration may be as often as twelve times daily to maintain therapeutic blood levels. The frequency of administration can be decreased by delaying absorption from the site of administration by using less soluble preparations. High blood levels are not reached with these delay preparations but they are useful if the organism is sensitive. Procaine Penicillin Injection B.P. may give antibacterial blood levels for up to 24 hours after a single dose. It is often combined with benzylpenicillin so that high initial levels of penicillin are quickly reached (Procaine Penicillin Injection, Fortified, B.P.).

Similar preparations are benethamine penicillin and benzathine penicillin which can give significant blood levels for a week or more after a single dose.

It is also possible to block the excretion of penicillin via the renal tubules by drugs such as probenecid. This is no longer done as other methods of maintaining blood concentration are preferable.

2. *Destruction by stomach acid.* The use of coated tablets or antacids has not proved satisfactory, but the development of acid-resistant penicillins such as phenoxymethylpenicillin has overcome this disadvantage. They are discussed later.

3. *Resistance and antibacterial spectrum.* Penicillin is active against cocci, Gram-positive bacteria, and spirochaetes. It is inactive against Gram-negative bacteria, *M. tuberculosis*, rickettsia viruses and fungi.

Previously sensitive organisms may develop strains which are resistant. This occurs especially with the staphylococcus partly due to its ability to produce penicillinase, an enzyme which destroys penicillin. Some strains of gonococcus have also become moderately resistant.

The newer penicillins

Attempts have been made to overcome these disadvantages of benzylpenicillin, and great advances were possible once the nucleus of penicillin, 6-aminopenicillanic acid, was isolated. This nucleus is modified to form a whole range of semi-synthetic penicillins. Other penicillins have been isolated after feeding different substrates to the *Penicillium* cultures (Table VIII). None of these penicillins, however, have the effectiveness of benzylpenicillin against sensitive organisms.

1. *Acid-resistant penicillins.* These are suitable for oral administration and include phenoxymethylpenicillin (penicillin V), phenethicillin and propicillin. All have approximately the same antibacterial spectrum as benzylpenicillin (see ampicillin below) but none is as effective against susceptible organisms. They are all destroyed by staphylococcal penicillinase (see cloxacillin below). They vary somewhat in their potency and protein binding but phenoxymethylpenicillin is probably the most useful. It may be advisable at the start of treatment to give systemic benzylpenicillin as well, as these oral penicillins take some 4 hours to reach peak blood level.

2. *Broad spectrum penicillins.* Ampicillin is less effective than benzylpenicillin against most Gram-positive bacteria but is active against some Gram-negative bacteria such as shigella (bacterial

TABLE VIII. The penicillins

Name of Penicillin	Acid-resistant	Penicil-linase-resistant	Antibacterial Spectrum
Benzylpenicillin	No	No	Especially Gram-positive cocci but not salmonella, shigella, Esch. coli, M. tuberculosis
Procaine penicillin	No	No	Similar to benzylpenicillin
Benzathine penicillin	No	No	but absorption is delayed
Phenoxymethylpenicillin ⎤ Phenethicillin ⎬ Propicillin ⎦	Yes	No	Similar to benzylpenicillin but less potent
Ampicillin	Yes	No	Similar to benzylpenicillin but only $\frac{1}{4}$–$\frac{1}{2}$ as potent. Also destroys salmonella, shigella, haemophilus, proteus and most Esch. coli
Methicillin	No	Yes	Activity similar to benzyl-penicillin but only 1/150th potency
Cloxacillin	Yes	Yes	
Flucloxacillin	Yes	Yes	

dysentery), salmonella (typhoid and paratyphoid), *Haemophilus influenzae*, some strains of proteus and most *Esch. coli*. It is also acid resistant and so can be given by mouth as well as intramuscularly and intravenously but is destroyed by penicillinase.

Carbenicillin has a similar spectrum to ampicillin but is also active against *Pseudomonas aeruginosa* (unless penicillinase producing as carbenicillin is not resistant). Carbenicillin is not acid stable and so must be given parenterally. It is often used with gentamicin in the treatment of severe infections.

3. *Penicillinase-resistant penicillins*. Methicillin, flucloxacillin and cloxacillin are active against penicillinase-producing staphylococci. Both flucloxacillin and cloxacillin are acid resistant and can be given orally though the former drug is the more reliably absorbed. Methicillin is not acid resistant and must be given parenterally.

Though these substances are penicillinase-resistant, they are relatively ineffective when compared with benzylpenicillin for the treatment of non-penicillinase-producing organisms.

Penicillin side effects. Penicillin is the least toxic of antibiotics

266 PHARMACOLOGY

and acute toxic effects are never seen unless an excessive dose (more than 20000 units) is given intrathecally.

Penicillin is, however, likely to cause sensitivity reactions ranging from immediate anaphylactic shock to a delayed type with fever and skin eruptions. Previous exposure to penicillin is likely to cause sensitization which is especially common in nurses, doctors, dentists, and in people with a previous history of eczema and allergy. The use of penicillin in veterinary and farming practices may cause reactions, especially if it contaminates foodstuffs such as milk. The incidence of sensitivity is probably 1–10% of the general population and there seems to be a cross sensitivity to all penicillins probably associated with the 6-aminopenicillanic acid nucleus or various breakdown products especially penicilloylated proteins.

CEPHALOSPORINS

These substances were originally isolated from the mould *Cephalosporium acremonium* and comprise at least three antibiotics known as Cephalosporin C,N, and P. Cephalosporin C is very similar to penicillin and its nucleus, 7-aminocephalosporanic acid has been isolated, and semi-synthetic derivatives prepared such as cephaloridine which are resistant to penicillinase. They are inactivated by cephalosporinase (β-lactamase).

Cephaloridine. This antibiotic has a similar antibacterial spectrum to ampicillin and acts by inhibition of cell wall synthesis. It is also resistant to penicillinase. Cephaloridine is not well absorbed and must be given parenterally. It is rapidly distributed but does not pass into the cerebrospinal fluid. There is little or no plasma binding and it is rapidly excreted unchanged via the kidney and has to be given 2–3 times a day. It appears to have a low level of toxicity though may cause necrosis of the proximal kidney tubules. There is some cross-resistance to penicillin and, very rarely, there may be cross-allergenicity. Cephaloridine is useful in the treatment of staphylococcus or streptococcus in penicillin-sensitive patients. It may also be used for *Esch. coli* infections of the urinary tract.

Other cephalosporins include cephalexin and cephradine which can be given orally, and cephalothin which must be given parenterally. These do not appear to be nephrotoxic.

STREPTOMYCIN AND
OTHER ANTITUBERCULOSIS DRUGS

1. *Streptomycin*. This antibiotic is isolated from *Streptomyces griseus*. It is an aminoglycoside and closely related to the neomycin group of drugs (page 272). Being a strong base, absorption from the gut is negligible so it may be used for sterilization of the gut. When given intramuscularly, it is quickly absorbed and distributed throughout the extracellular fluid though only traces enter the cerebrospinal fluid unless the meninges are inflamed. The blood level remains high for several hours, and above the inhibitory concentration for sensitive bacteria for about 8 hours. It is excreted unchanged via the kidney and the presence of renal damage may cause excessive blood levels due to impaired excretion.

The major use of streptomycin is against *Mycobacterium tuberculosis*, though it is active against many other organisms. The mode of action is discussed on page 255. The emergence of resistant strains is a serious problem and because of this, streptomycin is never used alone in the treatment of tuberculosis. Streptomycin is a toxic drug and is painful on injection. It produces general feelings of malaise and is likely to cause sensitivity reactions. It can also cause degeneration of the vestibular part of the auditory nerve, causing giddiness. The occurrence of this vestibular degeneration seems closely related to the size of the dose and the duration of treatment or the presence of renal disease delaying excretion.

2. *Isoniazid* (isonicotinic acid hydrazide, INAH). This is a synthetic drug and is very active against tuberculosis. It is readily absorbed from the intestine and is distributed throughout the extracellular fluid and cerebrospinal fluid. It is excreted mainly via the urine.

Isoniazid is inactivated by acetylation and people are either slow or fast inactivators (i.e. a bimodal distribution) due to a genetically determined level of enzyme. The incidence is race dependent and slow inactivators are common in Caucasians (around 50%) and uncommon in Japanese and Eskimos (around 5–10%). Slow inactivators, due to the higher blood level of isoniazid which can result, are more liable to get toxic effects. These include mental disturbances and a peripheral neuropathy which responds to pyridoxine treatment.

3. *Sodium aminosalicylate (p-aminosalicylic acid, PAS)*. This drug is synthetic and has a bacteriostatic effect on *M. tuberculosis* by an antimetabolite action. It is readily absorbed, distributed and rapidly excreted via the urine. It can cause alimentary side effects, sensitivity reactions and hypothyroidism.

4. *Ethambutol*. This drug may replace sodium aminosalicylate or streptomycin and is absorbed orally and excreted in the urine unchanged. Its most important adverse effect is retrobulbar neuritis initially characterized by a reduction in visual acuity and loss of colour discrimination. Other side effects are not important and rare.

5. *Rifampicin*. This drug may be given orally and is very active against *M. tuberculosis*. Some 65% is excreted via the bile and the drug may also stain the urine, tears and sputum a bright brownish red. Rifampicin may cause hepatotoxicity and purpura. Thrombocytopenia, fever, flush and gastrointestinal upset have been reported.

6. *Thiacetazone*. The major advantage of this drug is cheapness which makes it useful for the poorer countries. It is given orally and may cause nausea, vomiting and rashes. Agranulocytosis and anaemia have also been reported.

The drug treatment of tuberculosis

The treatment of tuberculosis has to be over a prolonged period of months or years, and the emergence of resistant bacterial strains or drug toxicity is a great problem. These are minimized by the concurrent use of several or more of the standard (first line) drugs. Streptomycin, isoniazid and sodium aminosalicylate are classical combinations but ethambutol, rifampicin and thiacetazone are also used on the grounds of variations in sensitivity side effects or cheapness.

Other drugs are also available but these are usually used only if resistance develops to the standard drugs. These second line or reserve drugs include pyrazinamide, prothionamide, ethionamide, cycloserine, viomycin and capreomycin. They are usually much more toxic than the standard drugs.

CHLORAMPHENICOL

This antibiotic was originally produced by a mould (*Streptomyces venezuelae*) but is now synthesized. It is almost completely absorbed from the gut; widely distributed, and enters the cerebrospinal fluid, though a large part may be protein bound. It is mainly excreted via the kidney as the conjugated inactive form.

Chloramphenicol is bacteriostatic and is active against a wide range of organisms including haemophilus, salmonella, bordetella and rickettsia. The mode of action is discussed on page 255.

The toxicity of chloramphenicol is of argued importance and includes gastrointestinal disturbances ranging from anorexia, nausea, vomiting and stomatitis to a fulminating superinfection, though these are less likely to occur than with the tetracyclines. Immature babies (who cannot metabolize the drug) are likely to get toxic levels of the drug which may induce a fatal circulatory collapse (grey syndrome). By far the most disputed toxic effect is the occurrence of a marrow aplasia which results especially with prolonged or repeated doses. The quoted incidence of marrow aplasia varies from 1/500 to 1/100000 and this together with the other toxic effects of chloramphenicol has lead to the view that the drug should be reserved solely for severe illness for which no other treatment is available. These include typhoid, haemophilus meningitis and severe whooping cough.

TETRACYCLINES

These are a family of broad spectrum antibiotics with only minor differences. They are amphoteric substances of low solubility and are poorly absorbed especially if calcium or iron containing compounds are given at the same time. Adequate blood levels of the tetracyclines may usually be reached by giving them orally every six hours and they are distributed throughout the extracellular fluid but intravenous injection may be necessary to get high levels in the cerebrospinal fluid. They are excreted in the bile, though some 25% is excreted unchanged via the urine.

The tetracyclines are bacteriostatic and their mode of action is discussed on page 255. They have a very wide range of action and act against most Gram-positive and Gram-negative organisms, spirochaetes, rickettsia, some viruses (lymphogranuloma, psittacosis, trachoma), but not against proteus, fungi or pseudomonas. Drug resistance is slow to emerge but may do so if treatment is prolonged, and there will be cross-resistance with other tetracyclines.

The toxic effects include gastrointestinal upsets ranging from nausea, diarrhoea and stomatitis to a fulminating enteritis. The tetracyclines are selectively bound in growing bone and teeth as they chelate with calcium. This causes hypoplasia and staining of the teeth, and the use of tetracyclines should be avoided in children younger than seven and in the pregnant woman.

Types of tetracyclines

The vast numbers of these reflect the manufacturers' ingenuity in chemical construction but are not necessarily a therapeutic advance.

1. *Tetracycline, chlortetracycline, oxytetracycline.* These are the original tetracyclines and show only small differences.

2. *Methacycline, demethylchlortetracycline.* These have twice the *in vitro* potency of tetracycline, are better absorbed and attain higher and more prolonged blood levels and so need to be given less often. These advantages are largely offset by the greater protein binding.

3. *Lymecycline.* This is a tetracycline made soluble by combination with lysine. Lymecycline is better absorbed and can be given intramuscularly as it is less irritant. It is questionable whether it has marked advantages, though the gut symptoms may be less as it is so well absorbed.

MACROLIDE (ERYTHROMYCIN) ANTIBIOTICS

Erythromycin, spiramycin and oleandomycin are a group of very similar antibiotics, though the latter two are the less effective. Chemically they consist of a macrocyclic lactone ring to which different sugars are attached.

They have much the same range of action as penicillin and their major use was in the treatment of penicillin-sensitive patients or of penicillin-resistant staphylococcal infection. Erythromycin may be given orally but is destroyed by acid so is given either in enteric coated capsules or as an ester (e.g. erythromycin estolate), which is more acid resistant. The estolate is more toxic and can cause liver damage. Drug resistance is prone to develop quickly with erythromycin and there is usually cross resistance with other members of the group.

POLYPEPTIDE ANTIBIOTICS

These antibiotics differ from the others in structure, source and actions. There are a large number of them but they are used mainly as local applications due to severe toxic reactions when given systemically.

1. *Polymyxin.* This antibiotic comprises at least 5 polypeptides obtained from *Bacillus polymyxa* and lettered A–E. Polymyxin B is the least toxic and is used clinically as the sulphate. It is not absorbed orally but may be given by injection, when it is slowly excreted via the urine. It is very active against Gram-negative bacteria, pseudomonas and shigella, but proteus, Gram-positive bacteria, neisseria and fungi are resistant. Polymyxin B is used especially for pseudomonas meningitis or septicaemia and can also be used to sterilize the gut or for local application.

Colistin is polymyxin E and its antibacterial action is similar.

2. *Bacitracin.* This is composed of three peptides, A, B, C, from a culture of *Bacillus subtilis*. It is very active against Gram-positive cocci and neisseria. It is very toxic, not readily absorbed and used mainly for local application.

3. *Gramicidin.* This polypeptide is highly insoluble and is very toxic. It has a limited use for topical application and is active against various Gram-positive cocci and some fungi. It is one of the components of tyrothricin.

NOVOBIOCIN, FUCIDIN, VANCOMYCIN, RISTOCETIN

These antibiotics may be used for the treatment of penicillin-resistant staphylococci. Novobiocin and fucidin may be taken by mouth, but vancomycin and ristocetin are badly absorbed and irritant and must be given by injection. They are all very toxic and can cause renal damage and deafness.

NEOMYCIN, FRAMYCETIN, KANAMYCIN, PAROMOMYCIN

(The Aminoglycosides)

These antibiotics were isolated from soil bacteria of the *Streptomyces* and are chemically related to streptomycin, and resemble it in their general toxicity and antibacterial action. They are likely to cause damage to the kidney and the auditory nerve and are used systemically only if essential.

Neomycin, a complex of antibiotics, may be used to sterilize the gut and is also effective in the local treatment of skin infections. Framycetin is similar, being one of the components of neomycin (neomycin B). Paromomycin is of use in the treatment of amoebic dysentery (page 281).

NITROFURANTOIN, NALIDIXIC ACID

Nitrofurantoin. This synthetic antimicrobial is well absorbed orally but rapidly broken down in the liver and quickly excreted in the urine especially if this is acid. It is used against urinary infections especially if caused by *Esch. coli* or some proteus but not pseudomonas.

Nitrofurantoin is likely to cause gastric upsets, peripheral neuritis, pulmonary infiltration and eosinophilia. Haemolytic anaemia may occur in those with glucose-6-phosphate dehydrogenase deficiency (Mediterranean races, Negroes, Sephardic Jews).

Nalidixic acid. This has a similar spectrum to nitrofurantoin and is also used in urinary infections. It is active against the majority of Gram-negative organisms including some proteus but not pseudomonas. It is absorbed readily by mouth and rapidly excreted in the urine, partly unchanged and part active metabolites. Nalidixic acid acts against organisms by preventing incorporation of precursors into DNA though still allowing synthesis of RNA and protein.

It can cause nausea, rashes and central disturbances.

TREATMENT OF FUNGAL INFECTIONS

Fungi are usually resistant to antibiotics, but some compounds do have an antifungal action. In general, fungal infections may be local or systemic. Local infections are usually a type of ringworm (*Trichophyton, Microsporum, Epidermophyton*) and affect the nails, skin, and hair. Systemic infections are much rarer and are often secondary to other causes such as superinfection by organisms such as *Actinomyces, Candida, Cryptococcus* (torula), during the use of broad spectrum antibiotics.

1. *Griseofulvin.* This antibiotic is isolated from *Penicillium griseofulvum* and is selectively effective in dermatophyte infections of the skin, nails and hair, but is of no use in yeast infections or candidiasis.

Griseofulvin is taken orally and is of no use as a local application. It is quickly absorbed from the upper part of the gut, giving peak plasma levels in 6 hours and becomes widely distributed in the tissues. Griseofulvin appears to be taken up in newly formed keratin of the skin, hair, and nails, where it exerts its antifungal action. Treatment must be continued till the infected keratin is all shed, which takes a few weeks for infections of thin skin to a year or so for toe nails.

Side effects with griseofulvin appear only minor, but it should not be used in liver disease, porphyrinuria or pregnancy. It may also alter the prothrombin time and interfere with the giving of anticoagulants.

2. *Nystatin.* This antibiotic was isolated from *Streptomyces noursei* and has no effect on bacteria or dermatophytes but is extremely effective in the treatment of yeast infections such as *Candida.* These are commonly of the skin and the mucous membranes of the mouth and vagina, though systemic candidiasis does occur. Infection is usually secondary to some other cause (e.g. superinfection due to broad spectrum antibiotics).

Nystatin is most commonly used as a local preparation in the form of a powder, ointment or suppository but it may be given parenterally. Nystatin is also effective against *Aspergillus* which may be present in some otitis externa or as aspergillosis of the lung.

3. *Amphotericin B.* This polyene antibiotic is produced by *Streptomyces nodosus* and may be used for the treatment of yeast infections. It may be used topically or parenterally by the intravenous route.

4. *Other topical antifungal preparations.* There are a vast

number of these, largely traditional but useful. Compound Benzoic Acid Ointment B.P.C. (Whitfield's ointment) is of use in dermatophyte infections and, as it is sticky, will trap loose and infected tissue.

Magenta paint and gentian violet are messy, though effective in some cases. Zinc undecenoate is relatively ineffective, and the use of tolnaftate and pecilocin have not been shown to be superior to other preparations.

ANTIVIRAL DRUGS

Viruses are obligatory intracellular parasites with no growth or reproduction *in vitro* save in some very specialized laboratory techniques. Attempts to find antiviral drugs have not been very successful and their use is complicated as the virus reaches a peak titre before symptoms are observed, so a drug used to prevent viral replication is best used prophylactically rather than left till gross symptoms occur. There are a few agents which, whilst mainly in the developmental stage, do show promise of antiviral action.

1. *Idoxuridine.* This compound is a thymidine analogue and is preferentially incorporated in viral DNA producing non-infectious material. It is very toxic and cannot be used systemically save in desperation. It has proved of value in the local treatment of superficial virus infections such as herpetic ulceration of the cornea.

2. *Thiosemicarbazones.* Some thiocarbazones such as methisazone have a wide antiviral action against both DNA and RNA viruses though the use of methisazone has so far been restricted to DNA virus infections. Methisazone has been shown to reduce the chance of a smallpox contact developing the disease but not effective in established smallpox. It may also be of use in the treatment of vaccination reactions which involve the local development and extension of the vaccination site due to virus multiplication.

3. *Amantadine hydrochloride.* This substance inhibits some myxoviruses such as human influenza and para-influenza. It is also of use in the treatment of Parkinsonism (page 51).

4. *Interferons.* These are proteins with an antiviral action produced by cells stimulated by some viruses (and other organisms such as certain bacteria and protozoa). Interferons do not act directly on the invading virus but probably so change the ribo-

somes of the host cell that viral RNA cannot complex with them, and so viral multiplication is stopped though normal development of the host cell is possible. The antiviral action of interferons is very broad and they are effective against a wide range of unrelated viruses. They have, however, a narrow host specificity and have little activity save in cells of the same or closely related species to that in which they were produced. Administration of exogenous interferons seems to be poorly effective, perhaps due to difficulties of reaching the reactive site, and the development of substances which stimulate endogenous interferon production seems more promising.

5. *Human immunoglobulins.* Normal plasma contains antibodies to many diseases and these antibodies are contained in the gamma globulin. Human specific immunoglobulins (previously known as hyperimmune or convalescent gamma globulins) may abort some virus infections if given in the incubation period. They are in very short supply and should only be used in cases at special risk such as poliomyelitis or German measles in the pregnant woman.

6. *Immunological methods* (see Chapter 25). The use of prophylactic vaccination is of immense use in the prevention of viral infection but is efficacious only if given sufficient time before exposure to allow immunity to develop. Rabies is an exception due to the unusually long incubation period and immunization begun shortly after exposure can confer protection rapidly enough to prevent the invasion of the central nervous system.

REFERENCES

Garrod, L. P., Lambert, H. P. & O'Grady, F. (1973) *Antibiotic and Chemotherapy,* 4th edn. Edinburgh: Livingstone.

Robson, J. M. & Stacey, R. S. (eds.) (1968) *Recent Advances in Pharmacology,* 4th edn. pp. 411–428, 429–448. London: Churchill.

23 Chemotherapy III: Antiprotozoal, Antihelminthic and Other Antiparasitic Drugs

Man, like all animals, is subject to infestation by many parasites other than bacteria and viruses. These parasites include protozoa, worms, lice, fleas and the scabies mite. The necessity for treatment requires careful judgment as in some cases the drugs used cause more toxicity than the infection itself.

Helminthiasis, or infestation with worms, is the most common disease in the world and the worms responsible come from widely different species which vary in form, habitat, physiology and sensitivity to drugs. Worms may be classified as the nematodes, the trematodes and the cestodes. The nematodes include such worms as roundworm, hookworm, threadworm, whipworm, filaria and trichinella. The cestodes include the various tapeworms such as *Taenia saginata* and *T. solium*. The trematodes (or flukes) are related to the tapeworms and include the flukes causing schistosomiasis. Antihelminthic drugs are used to rid the body of worms, and are sometimes called vermicides if they kill the worm and vermifuges if they merely expel it from the body.

It should be realized that immigration, rapid international air travel and the world-wide 'package holiday' have made these diseases, previously classified as 'tropical', nowhere near as uncommon in the U.K. as they were.

MALARIA

Malaria is an infectious disease of world distribution caused by protozoa of the genus *Plasmodium* and transmitted from man to man by the bite of the anopheles mosquito. In some areas malaria is endemic and is a very serious problem, causing perhaps some million deaths each year. It is no longer a problem in the United Kingdom though may occur in people who have travelled to infected areas.

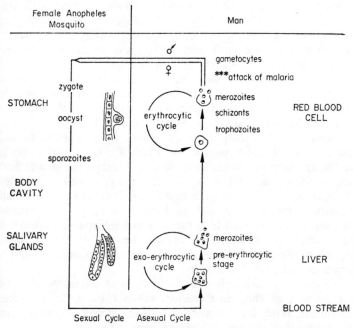

FIG. 14. The life cycle of the malarial parasite.

There are four species of *Plasmodium* pathogenic to man, all having a similar life cycle. They each cause a different and typical fever pattern, though mixed infections are not unknown. *P. vivax* causes benign tertian malaria in which fever occurs every 48 hours and is rather similar to that caused by *P. ovale* (ovale tertian malaria). *P. falciparum* causes the more serious malignant tertian (subtertian) malaria and *P. malariae* is responsible for the rare quartan malaria in which fever occurs every 72 hours. The diagnosis is made on the history and the demonstration of malarial parasites in the blood.

The life cycle of the malaria parasite

This is shown in Fig. 14. The female mosquito, by biting, injects sporozoites into the blood stream of the human host. These sporozoites rapidly accumulate in the liver and other reticulo-endothelial cells where they divide to form cyst-like structures which rupture to liberate merozoites (pre-erythrocytic cycle). The merozoites invade the red blood cells, though some (not in *P. falciparum* infections) may cause an exo-erythrocytic cycle to develop by invading other liver cells.

In the red blood cell the merozoites assume a ring-like shape (trophozoites) and divide (schizonts) to become merozoites, which are released along with foreign protein by rupture of the red cells to cause the clinical signs of the malarial attack.

Some of the erythrocytic merozoites develop into sexual forms, the male and female gametocytes, which if taken up by the bite of the appropriate anopheles mosquito, undergo the second and sexual side of their life cycle. The gametocytes become gametes in the stomach of the mosquito and fuse to become a zygote which penetrates the stomach wall to become an oocyst. Sporozoites develop in this oocyst which ruptures and releases them into the body cavity of the mosquito whence they invade most tissues, especially the salivary glands. They may then be injected into a new human host.

It is possible to interfere with this cycle at several points, but the control of the insect vector will not be discussed here. Obviously, however, this method is of the utmost importance in the eradication of malaria from an area.

Drugs used in Malaria

These have the three aims of prophylaxis, suppression and radical cure. The action of an antimalarial drug may be most effective at one stage or other during the life cycle of the parasite. A strict division is not possible, but it is helpful to group drugs according to their predominant use.

1. Drugs producing causal prophylaxis

These aim to prevent infection after the bite of an infected mosquito. A true causal prophylactic would kill the sporozoites in the blood stream of the human host before the start of the pre-erythrocytic stage. No drug, at present, does this, but it is possible to eliminate the parasite during the pre-erythrocytic stage. These drugs could be called tissue schizonticides.

(a) *Proguanil.* This drug is a biguanide and may be taken by mouth. It is completely absorbed but rapidly excreted and is metabolized in the body to an active form which probably suppresses nucleic acid synthesis in the malarial parasite by the inhibition of the conversion of folic acid to folinic acid (dihydrofolate reductase inhibitor). This effect is enhanced by giving sulphonamides at the same time (see page 259).

Proguanil is very effective against the pre-erythrocytic stage of *P. falciparum* though less so against *P. vivax.* It has no direct action on the gametocytes but, if carried over into the mosquito, will prevent the development of the sporozoite and thus prevent the mosquito becoming infected and spreading the disease. Proguanil is effective in an acute attack of malaria but is slow of action, and other drugs, such as chloroquine, are preferable.

(b) *Pyrimethamine.* This drug, a diaminopyrimidine, resembles proguanil in structure and acts similarly.

(c) *Trimethoprim.* This drug is also similar but has a greater activity on bacterial enzyme and is used in combination with sulphamethoxazole for bacterial infections (see page 262).

Prophylactic measures in malaria. It is advisable for all those entering or living in areas where malaria is endemic to take prophylactic measures which include avoidance of the mosquito (e.g. sleeping nets) as well as the taking of drugs. Both proguanil and pyrimethamine may be used as prophylactic drugs, though they provoke the emergence of resistant strains. Pyrimethamine needs to be taken only weekly when used as a prophylactic, and is the drug of the first choice but proguanil must be taken daily.

Chloroquine and amodiaquine, which are discussed below, may also be used as prophylactics. They will suppress all types of malaria and, as they are rapidly absorbed yet slowly excreted, a weekly dose is sufficient. Some forms of plasmodium resistant to chloroquine and amodiaquine have been reported, but are rare and occur mainly in the Far East and South America.

2. Suppressive drugs

These drugs or schizonticides inhibit the erythrocytic stages of *Plasmodium* and so stop the clinical signs of the disease and prevent symptoms. They do not destroy the exo-erythrocytic forms and so do not produce a radical cure save with *P. falciparum*, where there is no persistent exo-erythrocytic form. This persistence of the exo-erythrocytic stage may cause a relapse of clinical malaria once the suppressive therapy is stopped.

(a) *Quinine.* Quinine is an alkaloid extracted from Cinchona bark (Jesuit's bark) and has long been known as a cure for malaria. Quinine, which is only one of the twenty or so alkaloids present in the bark, is composed of a quinoline and a quinuclidine group joined by a secondary alcohol. It is laevorotatory, whilst its isomer, quinidine, is dextrotatory and has less antimalarial action (page 144).

The main action of quinine is on the erythrocytic forms of *Plasmodium,* but it is toxic and is now used only for those organisms resistant to other drugs. It is also used by intravenous infusion in the treatment of cerebral malaria.

The toxic symptoms or cinchonism include tinnitus, deafness and optic neuritis. Quinine idiosyncrasy may occur to cause collapse, skin eruptions and blackwater fever (haemoglobinuria due to intravascular haemolysis).

(b) *Chloroquine.* This drug (and the closely related amodiaquine) is a 4-aminoquinoline derivative. It is very effective against the erythrocytic forms of *Plasmodium* and quickly controls the clinical attack. It is rapidly absorbed by mouth but slowly excreted, being bound to plasma protein. It accumulates in the liver and exerts an appreciable effect against the hepatic forms of *Entamoeba histolytica* (page 281).

Chloroquine is relatively well tolerated though chronic administration of large doses (as may be given in rheumatoid arthritis) can cause reversible corneal opacities or a progressive and irreversible retinal pigmentation and damage which may lead to blindness.

(c) *Mepacrine* (*quinacrine*). This drug is a 9-amino acridine derivative and is very effective against the erythrocytic forms of most plasmodia. It may be given by mouth but can cause gastric upsets, central nervous depression or excitement. It also stains the skin yellow and is now little used, but may be effective in the treatment of tapeworm.

(d) *Proguanil and pyrimethamine*. These can be used for the suppression of clinical attacks of malaria but are slow to act (page 279).

3. Drugs producing radical cure

These drugs eradicate both erythrocytic and exo-erythrocytic forms of *Plasmodium*. They may also inactivate gametocytes.

(a) *Primaquine*. This 8-aminoquinoline derivative has both gametocidal action as well as destroying exo-erythrocytic forms. It has little schizonticidal activity and so is used in combination with chloroquine.

Primaquine may cause nausea, vomiting and abdominal pain. It can cause methaemoglobinaemia and intravascular haemolysis especially in dark-skinned races due to a genetically determined lack of glucose-6-phosphate dehydrogenase which makes the red cell fragile.

(b) *Pamaquin*. This is also an 8-aminoquinoline derivative but is more toxic than primaquine which has largely replaced it.

AMOEBIC DYSENTERY (AMOEBIASIS)

Amoebic dysentery is an acute or chronic infection caused by the protozoon *Entamoeba histolytica* and characterized by invasion of the mucous membrane of the large intestine with discharge of blood and mucus. It may also give rise to abscesses in the liver. Under adverse conditions (as when in faecal masses), the amoebae become cysts which can survive outside the body for a week or so in cool moist surroundings. These cysts can be transmitted by contamination with infected stools or via flies to cause new infections.

The treatment of amoebic dysentery may be considered as the suppression of the acute dysentery; the eradication of cysts; the treatment of liver abscess.

1. *Emetine hydrochloride*. This drug is an alkaloid isolated from ipecacuanha and is quickly effective in the suppression of acute amoebic dysentery.

It is given subcutaneously as it is very irritant by the oral route and causes vomiting and diarrhoea. Emetine is slowly eliminated and has a well-marked cumulative action. It is very toxic and can cause hypotension and heart damage, so careful hospital supervision is essential during treatment. If continued beyond 10 to 12 days it may cause localized peripheral neuritis with paralysis. Dihydroemetine is very similar to emetine but is probably less toxic.

Emetine completely eradicates the infection in only 10–30% of cases and the rest may become chronic and perhaps symptomless carriers.

2. *Emetine and bismuth iodide*. This can be given by mouth and will also kill amoebae in the lumen of the bowel.

3. *Diloxanide furoate*. This synthetic amoebicidal drug is given by mouth. It is active against amoebae in the bowel lumen and in chronic cyst-passing states to give about a 95% cure rate.

4. *Chloroquine*. This antimalarial drug is useless against intestinal amoebiasis but accumulates in the liver and may be effective in liver abscess.

5. *Metronidazole* (see below). This drug is effective in intestinal amoebiasis as well as the drug of choice in trichomoniasis.

6. *Antibiotics*. The tetracyclines are sometimes effective in chronic intestinal amoebiasis. Paromomycin, kanamycin, bacitracin and spiramycin may also be tried.

7. *Arsenicals*. The organic arsenical compounds have been used in the treatment of intestinal amoebiasis especially the less toxic pentavalent arsenicals such as carbarsone and glycobiarsol.

8. *Iodinated 8-hydroxyquinolones*. These drugs such as chiniofon, di-iodohydroxyquin and clioquinol (iodochlorhydroxyquin, Entero-Vioform) may also be used in intestinal amoebiasis. Clioquinol has a popular reputation as a prophylactic and treatment of mild infective enteritis.

TRICHOMONIASIS

Trichomonas vaginalis is one of the commonest causes of vaginitis, characterized by a severe pruritus and a creamy frothy discharge. It is diagnosed by inspection of the unstained wet smear or by culture. *T. vaginalis* is an ovoid, motile, flagellated parasite infecting some 20% of women and 2–10% of men. Non-symptomatic carrier states are common. The method of infection is usually venereal and both sexual partners need to be treated to avoid reinfection.

1. *Metronidazole*. This drug is given orally and cures up to 90% of cases. It perhaps should not be given during pregnancy to avoid risk of foetal damage, and is also excreted via the milk. Metronidazole is also used to treat amoebic dysentery.

2. *Local treatment*. This is not often required but includes the use of acetarsol, carbarsone or mercurial pessaries; or the painting of the vagina with antiseptics such as mercurochrome.

TRYPANOSOMIASIS

Trypanosomiasis is an infection caused by protozoa of the genus *Trypanosoma* carried by insect vectors of the genus *Glossina* (tsetse fly) from man and cattle. The trypanosomes are found in two forms. In the early stage of the disease, the blood contains the free-swimming flagellated trypanosome which later invades the lymph glands and the central nervous system to cause the characteristic depression which is ultimately fatal.

Sleeping sickness is caused by *T. gambiense* and *T. rhodesiense*, and Chagas' disease is caused by *T. cruzi*.

1. Arsenical compounds

Both pentavalent and trivalent arsenicals are actively trypanocidal though only the latter are active *in vitro* and the pentavalent arsenicals have to be reduced to the trivalent form *in vivo*.

(a) *Tryparsamide*. This pentavalent arsenical is very active and readily passes the blood–brain barrier and so is effective against trypanosomes in the central nervous system.

(b) *Melarsoprol*. This is a trivalent arsenical effective against central nervous infections. It is given intravenously.

(c) *Melarsonyl*. This is a water-soluble derivative of melarsoprol and is less toxic though still active against central nervous forms of the trypanosomes. It is given subcutaneously or intramuscularly.

2. Diamidines

Pentamidine is an aromatic diamidine and highly active, though not against the central nervous forms of the trypanosomes as it does not pass the blood–brain barrier.

It is used as a prophylactic and one intramuscular injection every 3–6 months gives protection.

3. Suramin

This drug is very effective against trypanosomes, though not the central nervous forms. It was used as a prophylactic but has been largely replaced by pentamidine.

LEISHMANIASIS

Leishmaniasis is an infection with protozoa of the genus *Leishmania* which are transmitted by the sandfly. These protozoa occur in the reticulo-endothelial system and give rise to many different forms of the disease.

L. donovani causes kala-azar; *L. brasiliensis* causes espundia; *L. tropica* causes cutaneous eruptions such as oriental sore.

Drugs used in leishmaniasis are the organic antimony compounds such as sodium stibogluconate, but pentamidine is also effective.

ROUNDWORM

This nematode (*Ascaris lumbricoides*) lives in the intestine where the female lays eggs. These are passed out in the faeces and eventually swallowed by another human lost. Larvae develop and penetrate the wall of the intestine to travel to the lung and then on, via the trachea and oesophagus, to reach the intestines as worms.

Piperazine. This is the drug of choice and hyperpolarizes the muscles of the worms thus paralysing them. They may then be expelled from the gut perhaps with the help of a purge. A single dose of piperazine (as the citrate, adipate or tartrate) is usually sufficient either in liquid or tablet form. Other drugs used are hexylresorcinol, bephenium hydroxynapthoate and diethyl-carbamazine.

THREADWORM (PINWORM)

Infection with threadworms (*Enterobius vermicularis*) is common though often symptomless apart from perianal itch (customarily at night).

Eggs are swallowed by the human host and hatch in the intestine into adult worms which have a life span of 2 months. They mate in the caecum and the female emerges from the rectum at night to lay eggs on the perianal skin. These eggs are mature in 6 hours but can survive for several days on the skin and up to 3 weeks in dust and bed-clothes.

Treatment must include appropriate hygiene measures to avoid reinfection (without which the worms would all die out in 2 months) and should include all members of the family.

1. *Piperazine.* This may be taken as a single dose followed by a saline or senna purge or preferably as a course lasting a week or so.

2. *Viprynium embonate.* This drug is used as a single dose and repeated after several weeks. It has the disadvantage of being more toxic than piperazine and can cause nausea and vomiting which is made aesthetically worse as viprynium is a red stain. It will also colour the stools red.

HOOKWORM

The two main pathogenic species of hookworm (*Necator americanus, Ancylostoma duodenale*) have a similar life history. They attach themselves to the mucosa of the intestine and feed on blood to cause severe anaemia, debility and malnutrition of the host.

The hookworms lay eggs which pass out in the faeces and develop into the infective stage in the soil to penetrate the intact skin of a new host and travel to the gut via the blood vessels, lungs and pharynx.

1. *Tetrachloroethylene.* This may be taken as an emulsion or in a capsule after a night of starvation and a saline purge. The purge is repeated two hours after the tetrachloroethylene, which can cause nausea, vomiting and diarrhoea.

2. *Bephenium hydroxynaphthoate.* This is preferable to tetra-chloroethylene as it is less toxic. It is also active against roundworms.

FILARIASIS

This is a systemic infection with nematodes of the family filariae. The adult worms (*Wuchereria, Brugia*) live in the lym-phatics where they cause obstruction which may become chronic to give the clinical picture of elephantiasis. Some species (*Loa, Onchocerca*) live in the subcutaneous connective tissue. The adult worms mate and the female lays free-swimming embryos (microfilariae) which live in the circulation by day and spend the night in the lungs. Infection is carried by a vector mosquito.

1. *Diethylcarbamazine.* This is a piperazine derivative and may be taken by mouth. It inhibits reproduction in the adult worm and rapidly clears the blood of microfilariae which go to the liver where they are phagocytosed or (*Onchocerca*) go to the skin where they are destroyed.

2. *Suramin.* This drug (which is also a trypanocide) has a marked effect on the adults of *Onchocerca* but not other filariae.

TAPEWORMS (CESTODES)

There are many kinds of tapeworms, some of which have a very complex life cycle. *Taenia saginata* (beef tapeworm) is the most common tapeworm in Britain. *Taenia solium* is found in measly pork.

1. *Dichlorophen.* This drug is effective and given in divided doses over 24 hours. The worm is expelled in a partially digested state and the head will not be found, so the stools of the patient should be examined 8 weeks later to see if treatment was successful.

2. *Felix mas.* This is an extract from rhizomes of male fern (*Dryopteris filix-mas*) of which filicic acid is the active principle. The patient is starved for several days and given a saline purge followed by the drug. The purge is repeated 2 hours later and the faeces examined for the head of the worm.

3. *Mepacrine.* This synthetic antimalarial drug is given as a single dose after preliminary starvation for 24–48 hours and followed by a saline purge after 2 hours. It may cause vomiting and a yellow staining of the skin.

TREMATODES

These worms (flat worms) have a very complex life cycle and some are pathogenic to man.

Schistosomiasis

The flukes *Schistosoma haematobium, S. mansoni, S. japonicum* live in the blood vessels of the gut and bladder. They lay eggs which, via the urine, infect the intermediate host, a species of water snail. Free-swimming larvae (cercariae) are released from the snail to infect the human host. Apart from general measures, such as sanitation and snail control, several drugs are of use.

1. *Antimony sodium tartrate.* This drug is very effective and given intravenously. It may cause nausea and vomiting and is also very toxic to the liver, kidneys, central nervous system and the heart.

2. *Niridazole.* This drug is less effective against *S. mansoni* than against *S. haematobium*. It may cause gastrointestinal upsets and cardiotoxicity. Niridazole also has some action against *E. histolytica*.

SCABIES

Scabies is a fairly common condition in Britain and is caused by a mite, *Sarcoptes (Acarus) scabiei*. The burrowing of the parasite into the skin causes widespread itching especially along the fingers, wrists, penis and breast, often with secondary eczema.

Various applications are used to kill the scabies mite.

1. *Benzyl benzoate.* This, used as a 25% emulsion, is effective but irritant and has a somewhat offensive smell.

2. *Gamma benzene hexachloride (gamma BHC)*. This may be used as a 1% cream and is very effective, non-irritant and has no smell. The B.P.C. formulation (Gamma Benzene Hexachloride Application) is 0·1% and not strong enough.

3. *Crotamiton.* This is used as a 10% lotion or cream.

4. *Monosulfiram.* 25% solution.

PEDICULOSIS

This is diagnosed by the presence of lice or ova (nits) in the hair (*Pediculus capitis*), body (*Pediculus corporis*), or pubic region (*Phthirius pubis*).

1. *DDT (dicophane)*. This may be used as a 10% powder which will have residual effects for weeks if left in the clothing. Some strains of *P. corporis* are resistant (see also page 112).

2. *Gamma benzene hexachloride (gamma BHC)*. This has a rapid action, though there is little residual effect. It is used as a cream, dusting powder or shampoo.

3. *Malathion*. This drug is not only an ovicide but has a marked residual action. It should be used only by trained persons.

REFERENCES

Bueding, E. & Swartzwelder, C. (1957) Anthelminthics. *Pharmacological Reviews*, **9**, 329.

Peters, W. (1968) Chemotherapeutic agents in tropical diseases. In *Recent Advances in Pharmacology*, 4th edn. Robson, J. M. & Stacey, R. S. (eds.). pp. 503–37. London: Churchill.

24 Chemotherapy IV: Cytotoxic Drugs

Cancer is characterized by cells which have undergone some fundamental and irreversible change which leads to their continuous and apparently unrestrained proliferation. This proliferation, eventually, will so interfere with body functions as to cause death.

The ultimate cause of cancer is not known though there is obviously a breakdown in the normal response to environmental and regulatory mechanisms for orderly cell development and integration.

Although surgery and irradiation techniques are still the mainstay of cancer treatment, great progress is being made in the use of chemical agents (cytotoxic drugs). These drugs prevent the growth and division of both normal and malignant cells and they are therefore of use only when the malignant cells exhibit enough qualitative differences to make them relatively sensitive enough and slow to recover. They are of most use in diseases like Hodgkin's disease, chorioncarcinoma, the Burkitt lymphoma, and various leukaemias. They are of much less value in bronchial, intestinal and breast cancer. Chemotherapy is often used in association with other procedures such as radiotherapy or excision. Save perhaps with chorioncarcinoma, it is rarely curative but will often produce prolonged remission or decrease the disability caused by the malignant tissue.

Complete eradication of all the tumour cells is desirable but is made difficult by the sensitivity of some normal cells to cytotoxic drugs. It is often possible to get better results by a combination of drugs having different modes of action so that the antitumour potential is increased without a parallel increase in toxic effects.

As the malignant cell and the normal cell may divide at different rates, it may be possible by the timing of dosage schedules to allow recovery of normal stem cells but to continue to depress malignant cells.

Cancer cells can also develop resistance to the cytotoxic drugs due either to the natural evolution of the tumour or to selective survival of pre-existing resistant cells and resistant mutant cells. As the general toxicity of the drug for the host remains unimpaired, the therapeutic ratio becomes even narrower. The role of immunological factors in cancer is also uncertain and the body seems to have no general mechanisms for disposing of even a few surviving cancer cells. This is in contrast to infectious disease where cellular, local and humoral defence mechanisms can dispose of large populations of micro-organisms.

Types of Cytotoxic Drugs

Some of these may be given by mouth, though some are so irritant that they must be given intravenously. Some cytotoxic drugs are given by intra-arterial perfusion which permits a selective concentration in the region of malignancy.

1. Biological alkylating agents

These drugs introduce an alkyl radical to a suitable receptor group usually through a nitrogen, sulphur or oxygen atom. They damage the desoxyribonucleic acids of the cells and produce an inhibition of growth. They react directly with the nucleic acid bases and cause crosslinking at the N.7 position between guanine groups on the same or adjoining chains.

(a) *Nitrogen mustards.* Mustine, mannomustine, trimustine, melphalan, chlorambucil and cylophosphamide.

(b) *Ethyleneimines.* Triethylenemelamine, triethylene thiophosphoramide.

(c) *Diepoxides.* Ethoglucid.

(d) *Dimesyloxyalkanes (alkyl methane sulphonates).* Busulphan.

(e) *Halogenated sugars.* Dibromomannitol.

The alkylating agents show much overlap in their actions and differ mainly in their solubility, stability and absorption. Busulphan has some preferential action on granulopoietic cells (e.g. myeloid leukaemia). The alkylating agents are of value in the treatment of Hodgkin's disease, chronic lymphocytic leukaemia, myelomatosis and ovarian adenocarcinoma.

The major toxic effects are bone marrow suppression, anorexia, nausea, vomiting and alopecia.

2. Antimetabolites

These cytotoxic drugs are structural analogues of substances essential for the synthesis and incorporation of constituent amino acids, purines and pyrimidines into nucleic acids. These analogues are of the following kinds:

(a) *Folic acid antagonists.* These drugs block the action of folic acid reductase which reduces dihydrofolic acid to tetrahydrofolic acid (essential for the biosynthesis of purines and pyrimidines).

Methotrexate is the most commonly used folic acid antagonist and is of value in the treatment of lymphoblastic leukaemia and chorioncarcinoma. Folinic acid (formyltetrahydrofolic acid), the active form of folic acid, may be used as a specific antidote to methotrexate as its action is not affected by the block of folic acid reductase.

(b) *Purine and pyrimidine antagonists.* These interfere with the normal synthesis of the nucleic acids. They may be purine analogues such as 6-mercaptopurine, which is effective in the treatment of acute lymphoblastic leukaemia and chorioncarcinoma. Azathioprine is a derivative of 6-mercaptopurine used mainly as an immunosuppressive agent (page 299).

Fluorouracil is a pyrimidine analogue active against carcinomas of breast, stomach, rectum and ovary.

3. Natural substances

(a) *Antibiotics.* Many streptomyces or related organisms produce substances which can be used as cytotoxic drugs. These include actinomycin D which interferes with the replication processes of DNA (page 255). Other similar substances are mitomycin C and puromycin.

(b) *Colchicine*. This drug is obtained from *Colchicum autumnale* and arrests mitosis at metaphase. It may also be of use in the treatment of acute gout (page 178).

(c) *Vinca alkaloids*. Alkaloids such as vinblastine and vincristine have been isolated from the periwinkle (*Catharanthus roseus, Vinca rosea*). They arrest mitosis at the metaphase and are of use in the treatment of Hodgkin's disease and lymphoblastic leukaemia.

(d) *Asparaginase*. Some tumour cells (e.g. lymphoblastic leukaemia and reticulum cell sarcoma) have lost the normal ability to synthesize the amino acid asparagine though it is necessary for their metabolism.

L-Asparaginase isolated from guinea-pig serum and from some strains of *Esch. coli*, and *Erninia carotovera* breaks down asparagine to aspartic acid and so deprives the tumour cells of asparagine. Normal cells are not affected as, for them, asparagine is not essential.

(e) *Hormones*. Some tumours may be hormone dependent and changing the hormonal environment may cause regression of the tumour.

Some premenopausal carcinomas of the breast, for example, are oestrogen dependent, and may regress if endogenous secretion of oestrogens is reduced to a minimum. Methods employed include oophorectomy, adrenalectomy and pituitary ablation.

Many carcinomas of the prostate, on the other hand, are androgen dependent and production of these hormones may be reduced by castration or by giving oestrogens.

The lympholytic actions of the corticosteroids (page 108), such as prednisone, makes them useful in lymphoid neoplasms.

However, hormonal treatment of carcinoma has many unresolved problems; one of which is to identify the patient who will benefit. It is unfortunate that, whilst hormones may cause regression of some carcinomas, they may stimulate the growth of others which are apparently similar.

4. Radio-active Compounds

Ionizing radiation is cytotoxic and radioactive isotopes have been used.

Radio-gold (^{198}Au) has a half-life of 2·7 days and can be injected in peritoneal and other cavities to treat malignant effusions.

Radio-phosphorus (^{32}P) has a half-life of 14·3 days and, although normal tissues have a high uptake, concentrates in bone and is used to treat chonic leukaemias and polycythaemia vera.

Radio-iodine. There are several isotopes of iodine used therapeutically. ^{131}I has a half-life of 8 days and is rapidly taken up by the thyroid and is used to treat hyperthyroidism (page 128) but is not so successful in thyroid carcinoma which may not take up iodine well. ^{132}I has a short half-life (2⅓ hours) and is used as a tracer in metabolic studies of the thyroid.

REFERENCES

Boesen, E. & Davis, W. (1969) *Cytotoxic Drugs in the Treatment of Cancer.* London: Arnold.

Cooper, E. H. & Amiel, J. J. (1968) The immunosuppressive drugs. In *Recent Advances in Pharmacology*, 4th edn. pp. 449–78. Robson, J. M. & Stacey, R. S. (eds.). London: Churchill.

The body has elaborate mechanisms for defence against micro-organisms which involve the production of antibodies. These antibodies are found mainly in the plasma gamma globulins and are formed by the spleen, lymph nodes and bone marrow in response to the injection of an antigen. The general term antigen is used to describe any substance which elicits the formation of antibodies and is often a micro-organism or its products.

The antigen and antibody react in several ways. They may form lattices of antigen–antibody complexes which precipitate; the antibodies may cause clumping of bacteria, make them susceptible to phagocytosis by white cells or dissolve them. These mechanisms contribute to the immunity to infection which is the ability of the body to resist invasion by micro-organisms.

The immunity is very specific for the micro-organism (i.e. the particular protein complex) involved and is often acquired during the course of an infection. This infection may be either a florid form or a subclinical form which, whilst symptomless, is adequate enough in antigenic effect to promote an immune response. This immunity aids the body to combat a repeat infection and persists for a variable period; perhaps for life after smallpox or very transiently with influenza.

The immunological response may be used in the diagnosis, prevention and treatment of many diseases.

Diagnostic Procedures

These include the Mantoux test in which a purified tuberculo-protein (tuberculin) is given intradermally either by injection or the multiple puncture technique (Heaf test). If the subject has been previously exposed to tuberculosis (and so will not gain from active immunization with BCG), erythema and induration will be present at the inoculation site within 48–72 hours.

Other diagnostic tests include the Schick test for scarlet fever and the Dick test for diphtheria, in which a small amount of the specific toxin is injected intradermally. If the subject is susceptible, erythema appears around the inoculation site, usually within 24–48 hours though perhaps not for some days.

ACTIVE IMMUNIZATION

Immunity may be acquired artificially (active artificial immunity) by the giving of vaccines. These are preparations of antigenic material which may be suspensions of the living or dead organisms (bacteria or viruses). Vaccines may also be toxoids which are toxins so modified as not to produce the actual disease but still able to produce specific immunity to the particular organism. Active immunity must be distinguished from passive immunity (discussed below) as in active immunity the recipient is stimulated to produce his own antibodies and keeps this property for a variable time depending on the particular disease.

1. Smallpox Vaccine (Var/Vac)

This contains the living virus of vaccinia (cowpox) and is inoculated by multiple pressure or by scarification. In primary vaccination, this causes a vesicle to form in 5 days which becomes pustular and then forms a scab which separates in about 3 weeks. Mild reactions are common but there is also the danger of serious complications such as post-vaccinial encephalitis or generalized vaccinia.

Although protection may last for 5–7 years, the international Vaccination Certificate is valid for only 3 years and more frequent vaccination is advisable in countries where smallpox is endemic. Contacts of smallpox may be wholly protected by vaccination within 24 hours, but only partially so if within 3 days (see also Methisazone, page 274).

2. Poliomyelitis Vaccine

There are two kinds of these; the subcutaneous (Salk type) and the oral (Sabin type).

(a) *Poliomyelitis Vaccine (Inactivated)* (*Pol/Vac (Inact)*). This is an aqueous suspension of the formaldehyde inactivated viruses of the three main strains of poliomyelitis grown on monkey kidney. It is given subcutaneously or intramuscularly and provides good protection against the paralytic form of poliomyelitis but does not reduce the intestinal carriage of the virus.

(b) *Poliomyelitis Vaccine (Oral)* (*Pol/Vac (Oral)*). This is an aqueous suspension of the live attenuated virus grown on monkey kidney and has lost the capacity to invade the central nervous system. The vaccine may contain one strain of the virus (monovalent) or the three main strains (trivalent). It is given orally and provides good protection against the paralytic form of poliomyelitis as well as giving gut immunity.

3. Bacillus Calmette-Guérin Vaccine (Dried Tub/Vac/BCG)

BCG vaccine is a suspension of an attenuated bovine strain of tuberculosis and is used for the active immunization of people with a negative tuberculin reaction. It is given intradermally and provides substantial though not complete protection for 6 years or so.

4. Diphtheria Vaccine (Dip/Vac)

This vaccine is made from diphtheria toxin produced by *Corynebacterium diphtheriae* and is available in several forms.

(a) *Diphtheria Vaccine (Dip/Vac/FT)*.

(b) *Adsorbed Diphtheria Vaccine (Dip/Vac/Adsorbed)*

Diphtheria vaccine is used for active immunization against diphtheria. In primary immunization of young children, multiple vaccines are available containing combinations of vaccines against diphtheria, pertussis and tetanus, though the most used is Diphtheria, Tetanus and Pertussis Vaccine (DTPer/Vac).

5. Pertussis Vaccine (Per/Vac)

This is a sterile suspension of killed *Bordetella pertussis* and is used for active immunization against whooping cough. It is commonly used as one of the multiple vaccines.

6. Tetanus Vaccine (Tet/Vac)

This is prepared from tetanus toxin produced by the growth of *Clostridium tetani* and stimulates the production of tetanus antitoxin or increases the amount of antitoxin if already present. It is available in several single forms as well as in multiple vaccines.
   (a) Tetanus Vaccine (Tet/Vac/FT)
   (b) Adsorbed Tetanus Vaccine (Tet/Vac/Adsorbed)

7. Measles vaccine

This is available as Measles Vaccine (Live Attenuated). This vaccine is grown on chick embryos and should not be given to patients who are sensitive to egg protein.

8. Other vaccines

There are many other vaccines, and works of reference such as the *British Pharmacopoeia* and the *British Pharmaceutical Codex* should be consulted for details. They include vaccines against cholera, gas-gangrene, influenza, plague, rabies, scorpion venom, snake venom, staphylococcus, typhoid, paratyphoid, typhus and yellow fever. There are also combined vaccines which contain two or more simple vaccines and may be preferred when immunizing against several diseases.

PASSIVE IMMUNIZATION

Passive immunization may be brought about by the injection of the serum of an actively immunized man or animal and depends entirely on the antibodies or antitoxins produced by the donor during the active immunization. Passive immunization also occurs in the fetus due to maternal antibodies passing across the placenta.

Passive immunity is transient, lasting only a few weeks, as the transferred antitoxins and antibodies are soon eliminated by the recipient, especially if they have been given on a previous occasion. Administration of these antisera is therefore usually an emergency procedure and should be followed by steps to produce active immunity.

As these antisera may also contain foreign protein derived from the donor, reactions to them are common. These reactions range from serum anaphylaxis, an immediate and often fatal collapse, to serum sickness which occurs in 3–10 days accompanied by rashes, pyrexia and joint pains. It is advisable to enquire about previous history of allergy and to do a subcutaneous trial dose before injecting the main bulk of the antiserum.

Antisera may be antitoxic, antibacterial, or antiviral. Antitoxic sera are produced for use against diseases like diphtheria, tetanus, and gas gangrene, where the bacteria involved produce an exotoxin and the antiserum has the specific antitoxin to neutralize the toxin.

Some bacteria do not produce exotoxins and the antibacterial sera contain antibodies against the bacteria themselves to make susceptible to phagocytosis.

Antisera are also available for use against the viruses of measles, rubella, rabies and smallpox. They are in very short supply for they are obtained (save for rabies) from adults who have had the disease. Human immunoglobulin (previously called human gamma globulin) is prepared from pooled human plasma and is available for the prophylaxis of some common virus diseases such as measles, rubella, poliomyelitis and infectious hepatitis.

Immunization Schedules

Information on the giving of these immunological products can be found in the *British Pharmaceutical Codex*, the *British National Formulary* and the recommendations of the Department of Health and Social Security (1972).

IMMUNOSUPPRESSIVE DRUGS

These drugs are used to treat transplantation rejection reactions by a host to an allograft (a transplant from a different member of the same species). They may also be used to treat autoimmune disease which may be defined (Burnet) as '... Interaction within the body of antibody or immunologically competent cells on the one hand and antigenic determinants carried by the normal body components on the other.'

Most immunosuppressive drugs have well recognized anti-leukaemic or antitumour effects and are discussed elsewhere. They include the corticosteroids, folic acid antagonists, pyrimidine and purine analogues, alkylating agents and antibiotics such as actinomycin, mitomycin and puromycin.

Antilymphocytic sera (ALS). These sera are the most powerful immunosuppressive agents available and are formed by injecting heterologous lymphoid tissue into a suitable recipient animal which responds by making antibodies specific for the foreign lymphocytes. When these antibodies are injected back into the donor animal, they inactivate the donor lymphocytes which are responsible for cell-mediated immunity.

Although ALS is a highly specific immunosuppressive drug, recent work has shown that its use may predispose the recipient to cancer.

REFERENCES

British Medical Bulletin (1969) **25,** 2. Immunization against infectious disease.

Cooper, E. H. & Amiel, J. J. (1968) The immunosuppressive drugs. In *Recent Advances in Pharmacology*, 4th edn. pp. 449–78. Robson, J. M. & Stacey, R. S. (eds.). London: Churchill.

The British Pharmacopoeia.

The British Pharmaceutical Codex.

The British National Formulary.

Whilst systemic infections with micro-organisms are treated by systemic therapy, it may often be desirable to reduce or abolish the organisms present on surfaces ranging from the skin and mucous membranes to crockery, clothing and floors.

The nomenclature is confusing owing to loose popular usage. Sterilization means to cause the death of all contaminating life, but antiseptic and disinfectant are more equivocal. Some (correctly) restrict the term antiseptic to agents which destroy micro-organisms on living tissue and disinfectant to agents used on inanimate surfaces. The term skin disinfection is in common use, however. Germicide is a broad term and is an agent that destroys micro-organisms. It may be more specifically defined as a bactericide, fungicide or virucide.

Evaluation of antimicrobial activity. Germicidal action is a function of time, temperature, concentration of the germicide and the number and type of the infecting organisms as well as the presence of other substances such as blood and pus.

The original test (Rideal–Walker) was to compare the activity with that of phenol under standard conditions, but this test has many inadequacies. *In vitro* testing, on the whole, has failed to provide suitable comparative information. All micro-organisms are not equally easy to kill and it is important to know the range a particular germicide will destroy. It is usually easy to kill vegetative cells and some viruses such as rabies and influenza. The tubercle bacillus has a waxy coat which makes it resistant. The enteric viruses (poliomyelitis, echo, coxsackie) are not easy to destroy. Spores are extremely resistant and most of the normal germicides do not harm them.

Individual Germicides

Many substances are used for their germicidal action, though a large number are obsolete and are not discussed here. These include the heavy metals, boric acid and many dyes.

Ideally, a germicide should be effective in high dilution even in the presence of foreign proteins, exudate or other matter. It should not damage tissue or inanimate objects and should be stable, odourless, non-staining and inexpensive.

1. Alcohols

Both isopropyl and ethyl alcohol are efficient germicides. Ethyl alcohol is most effective in a 70% concentration when it will destroy vegetative cells, the tubercle bacillus, some viruses but not spores.

The alcohols are expensive and inflammable, which restricts their wholesale use. They are often used in combination with other germicides.

2. Surface-active agents

(a) *Soaps*. Normal soaps are bactericidal to some organisms such as pneumococcus but are relatively inert to others such as *Staph. aureus*. They are often combined with other germicides such as hexachlorophane.

(b) *Detergents*. These are long-chain molecules with a hydrophilic group at one end and a hydrophobic group at the other. They accumulate at interfaces between oils and water to lower the surface tension and so facilitate cleansing as well as destroying micro-organisms. They may be classified as anionic, cationic, or amphoteric according to the charge on the hydrophilic group.

The cationic detergents such as cetrimide, domiphen and cetylpyridinium (inverted soaps) are quaternary ammonium derivatives. They are both cleansing and rapidly bacteriostatic especially against Gram-positive organisms, though relatively ineffective against spores, tubercle bacillus and fungi. They are non-toxic and are used a great deal in washing-up liquids, though on occasion may cause sensitivity and allergic skin reactions.

They are inactivated by soaps, anionic detergents, organic matter and hard water. Hands absorb some 20 mg from a 1/1000 solution so, for germicidal purposes, a dispenser should be used and not a communal dip.

3. The halogens

(a) *Iodine and the iodophors.* Elemental iodine is an active germicidal agent though it is inhibited by the presence of reducing agents or organic material. It is active against Gram-positive and Gram-negative bacteria as well as many spores. It is also active against the tubercle bacillus, *cercaria, leptospira, E. histolytica,* fungi, yeasts and many viruses (though the enteroviruses may be resistant). Iodine is commonly used as a 2·5% solution in 70% alcohol (Weak Iodine Solution B.P.). Iodine has the disadvantage of being irritant and staining.

The iodophors such as povidone iodine are combinations of iodine and surface-active agents such as non-ionic detergents, quaternary compounds and macromolecules. Their detergent properties aid the cleaning and germicidal processes. The iodophors are non-irritant, non-toxic, non-staining, miscible with water, and act by slowly releasing iodine. They can be used for topical application, irrigation of mucous membranes and the disinfection of inanimate surfaces.

(b) *Chlorine.* Compounds releasing chlorine form excellent germicides but have the disadvantages of being quickly inactivated by protein and having a bleaching action.

(c) *Organic halogen compounds.* Halogenated derivatives of phenol and cresol have enhanced germicidal powers.

(i) Chlorocresol is added to multidose containers to preserve sterility.

(ii) Amyl-m-cresol, thymol: these compounds are used as gargles and preservatives.

(iii) Chloroxylenol is the basis of many proprietary compounds (e.g. Dettol, Roxenol) which, whilst pleasant smelling, have poor antibacterial power. They cannot be relied upon to destroy staphylococci.

(iv) Hexachlorophane is a chlorinated bisphenol linked by a methylene bridge. It is colourless, crystalline, very slightly soluble in water but soluble in alcohol and glycols. It has a slow-acting bacteriostatic action especially against *Staph. aureus* and skin micrococci but is relatively inactive against Gram-negative organisms. It is compatible with soap and leaves a germicidal residue on the skin which is removed by alcohol. It is non-irritating, relatively non-toxic and rarely causes allergic reactions. Hexachlorophane can be absorbed through the skin and cause c.n.s. toxicity which has caused deaths in babies. Its unrestricted use in newborn infants is inadvisable and it is essential to use the correct dilutions and methods.

(v) Chlorhexidine has a wide antibacterial action. It is non-irritant, non-toxic and is used in aqueous or alcoholic solution or as a cream.

4. Gas sterilization

It is often necessary to sterilize equipment which may be damaged by heating or the use of the usual germicides. It may be possible, in these circumstances, to use a germicidal gas.

(a) *Formaldehyde.* This is a powerful disinfectant in solution but may be used as a gas produced by heating the solid paraformaldehyde. Formaldehyde can be removed by ammonia which combines with it to form the inert solid, hexamine.

(b) *Ethylene oxide.* This substance (b.p. 10·7°C) is a gas at normal room temperatures. It is toxic, inflammable and forms explosive mixtures with air unless also mixed with an inert gas such as carbon dioxide. It is effective though slow in action.

Physical means of sterilization

These include the application of heat by boiling or autoclaving and the application of ultraviolet light or gamma radiation. The use of disposable equipment sterilized by gamma radiation and the provision of sterile packs of instrument by centralized units has revolutionized many surgical techniques.

'Scrubbing up'

The doctor is perhaps most personally concerned with the microflora of his own skin and methods of reducing it before using surgical techniques.

This microflora is of two kinds: actively growing resident colonists and transients. Whilst much of the resident flora is non-pathogenic. *Staph. aureus* may be present.

Simple scrubbing of the skin will practically abolish the transient population but will only reduce the resident flora to about half as these live deep in the follicles and crevices of the skin.

The resident flora may be more efficiently removed by the use of germicides and it is often convenient to incorporate these in a soap or detergent. Hexachlorophane is especially useful as it has a cumulative effect due to the residue left on the skin which, however, is removed by alcohol. It is available as various proprietary preparations of detergent creams, liquid soaps, and hard soaps. Hexachlorophane is relatively inactive against Gram-negative organisms but as these are mainly transients, they will be removed by a detergent.

Iodophors such as povidone iodine are quicker acting than hexachlorophane and also destroy Gram-negative organisms and some spores. Povidone iodine may also be applied as a compress, and soaking the skin for $\frac{1}{2}$–1 hour will kill the majority of spores in ingrained dirt.

REFERENCE

Kundsin, R. B. & Walter, C. W. (1968) Antiseptics and disinfectants. *Practitioner*, 200, 15.

Additional Reading

These are given so that the student may expand his knowledge of any desired topic. Further references have been given at the end of each chapter but are not intended to be exhaustive.

Goodman, L. S. & Gilman, A. (1975) *The Pharmacological Basis of Therapeutics*, 5th edn. Baillière Tindall: London, New York: Macmillan.

Barlow, R. B. (1964) *Chemical Pharmacology*, 2nd edn. London: Methuen.

Robson, J. M. & Stacey, R. S. (eds.). (1968) *Recent Advances in Pharmacology*, 4th edn. London: Churchill.

Holmstedt, B. & Liljestrand, G. (1963) *Readings in Pharmacology*. London: Pergamon Press.

Annual Reviews of Pharmacology
British Journal of Pharmacology
Journal of Pharmacology and Experimental Therapeutics
Prescribers' Journal

The British National Formulary
The British Pharmacopoeia
The British Pharmaceutical Codex
The Extra Pharmacopoeia: Martindale

Index